JUST THE BASICS COOKBOOK

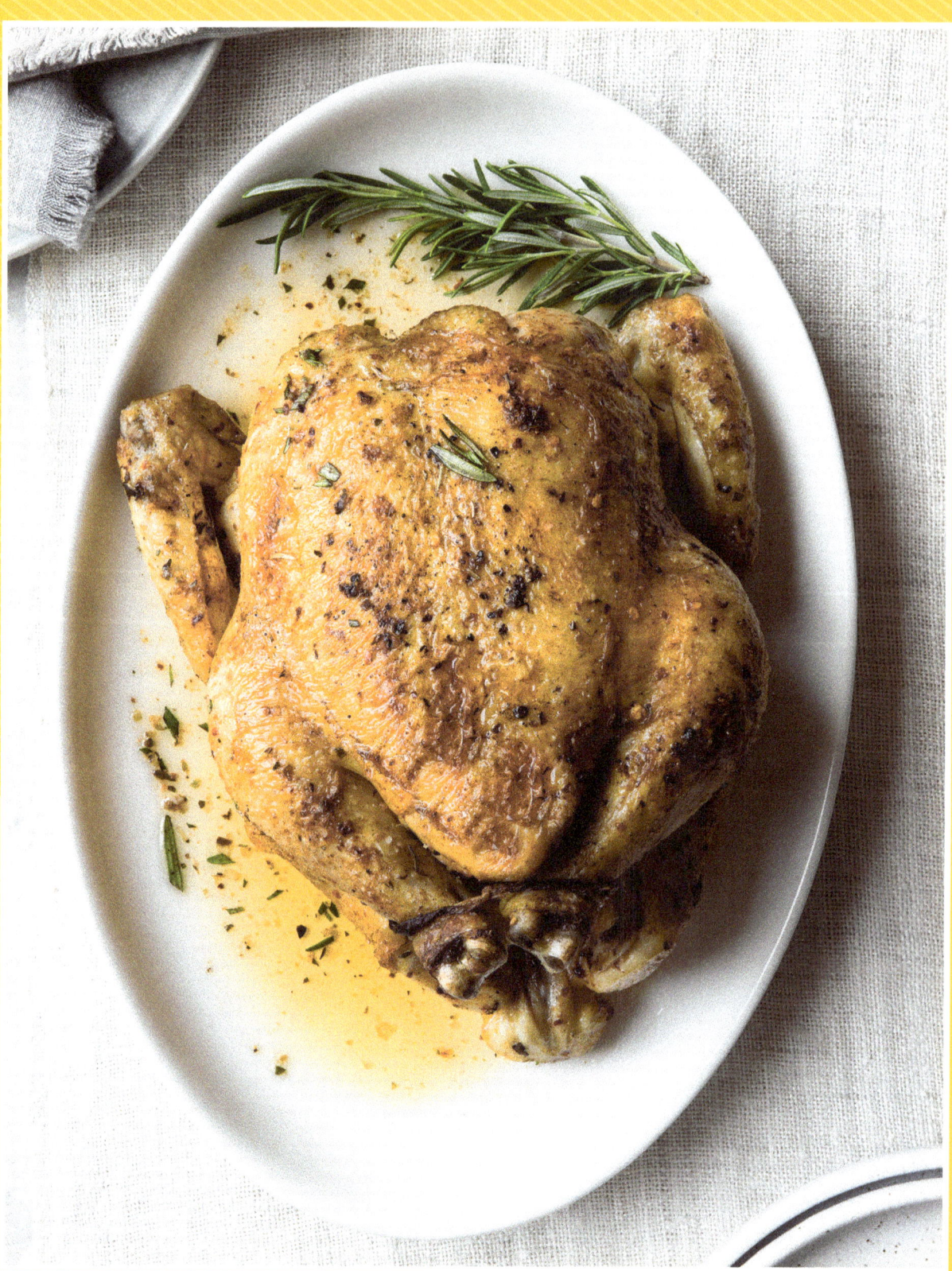
Perfect Roast Chicken, page 86.

JUST THE BASICS COOKBOOK

Learn How to Cook with Essential Techniques and Fundamental Recipes

CHRISTINA HITCHCOCK

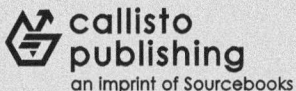

Copyright © 2022 by Callisto Publishing LLC
Cover and internal design © 2022 by Callisto Publishing LLC
Illustrations © Tom Bingham
Cover photo © Chaded Panichsri/Shutterstock; Nadine Greeff, ii, 72; Russel Brown/StockFood USA, vi; YoPho/Shutterstock, x; Eisling Studio/StockFood USA, 14; Sporrer/Skowronek/StockFood USA, 26; Alex Luck/StockFood USA, 44; Andre Baranowski/StockFood USA, 56; Profimedia/StockFood USA, 90; Kelly Knox/Stocksy United, 108; Marti Sans/Stocksy United, 128; Ina Peters/Stocksy United, 144
Interior and Cover Designer: Jennifer Hsu
Art Producer: Megan Baggott
Editor: Anne Lowrey and Cecily McAndrews
Production Editor: Caroline Flanagan
Production Manager: Martin Worthington

Callisto and the colophon are registered trademarks of Callisto Publishing LLC.

All rights reserved. No part of this book may be reproduced in any form or by any electronic or mechanical means including information storage and retrieval systems—except in the case of brief quotations embodied in critical articles or reviews—without permission in writing from its publisher, Sourcebooks LLC.

All brand names and product names used in this book are trademarks, registered trademarks, or trade names of their respective holders. Callisto Publishing is not associated with any product or vendor in this book.

Published by Callisto Publishing LLC C/O Sourcebooks LLC
P.O. Box 4410, Naperville, Illinois 60567-4410
(630) 961-3900
callistopublishing.com

Printed in the United States of America.

To all of my readers and *It Is a Keeper* fans.
Your continued support inspires me every day.

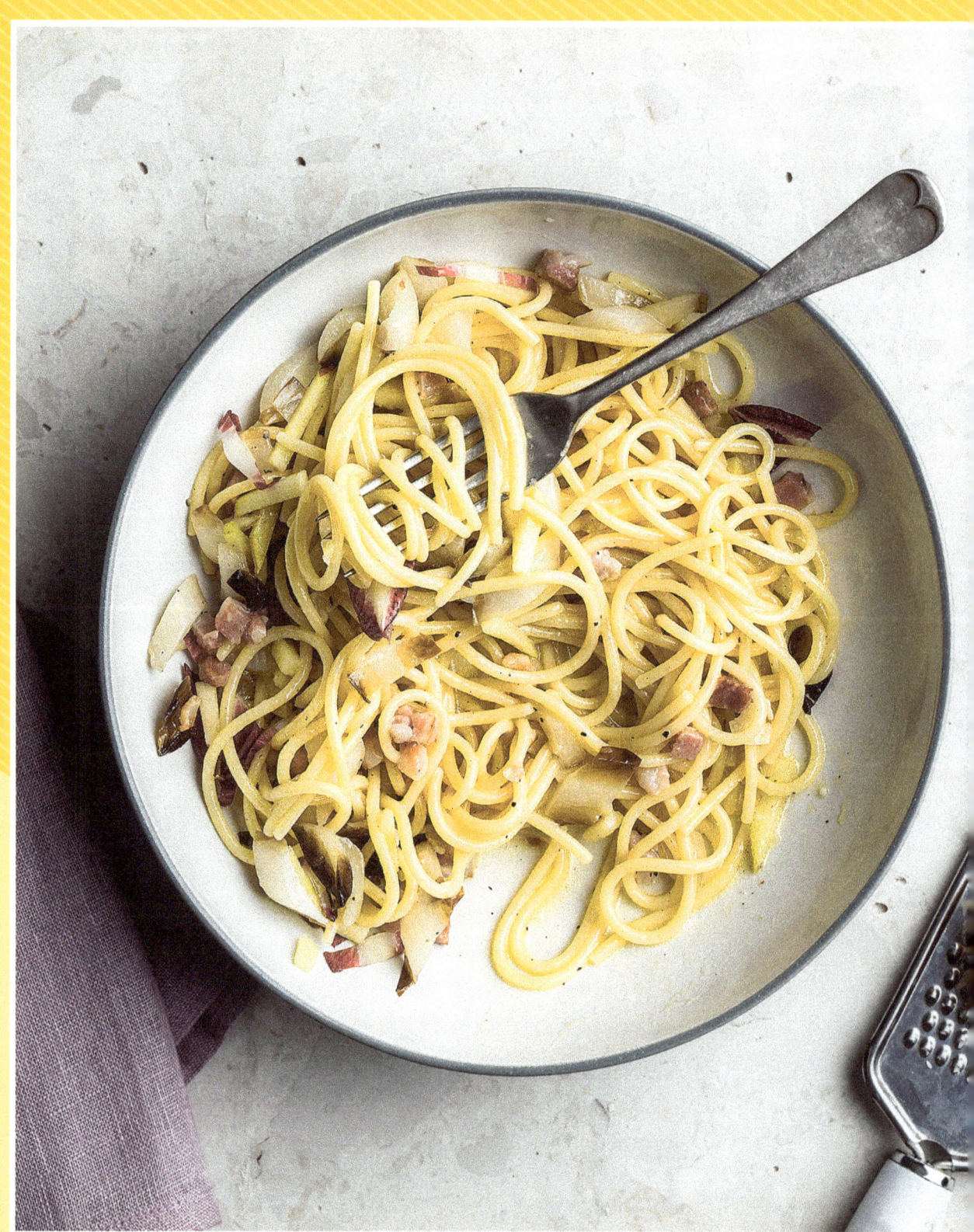

Velvety Pasta Carbonara, page 40.

Contents

INTRODUCTION viii

Chapter 1: **Kitchen Fundamentals** 1

Chapter 2: **How Flavor Develops** 15

Chapter 3: **Beans, Grains, and Pastas** 27

Chapter 4: **Fruits and Vegetables** 45

Chapter 5: **Seafood** 57

Chapter 6: **Eggs and Poultry** 73

Chapter 7: **Beef, Pork, and Lamb** 91

Chapter 8: **Sweet and Savory Baking** 109

Chapter 9: **Recipes That Bring It All Together** 129

MEASUREMENTS AND CONVERSIONS 145

RESOURCES 146

INDEX 147

Introduction

When I was growing up, my mom would often ask me to get dinner started while she was on her way home from work. I can remember standing over the stove wondering how I could coax more flavor out of a jar of marinara sauce. I would try adding a pinch of this or a splash of that. I didn't quite know what I was doing at the age of 12, but I loved experimenting with ingredients and flavors.

Fast-forward a few decades, and I now understand what goes into a great recipe. Over the years, I learned everything I could about flavors and techniques. I've spent a lot of time in the kitchen trying new recipes and experimenting with different ingredients. I made many mistakes, but I learned from them. And, more importantly, I kept cooking.

I often say that if you can read, you can cook. But it's really a little more involved than that. To make great-tasting food, you need to understand how to build flavor and balance ingredients. It also helps to learn proper technique so you're more efficient when cooking.

This book will show you what you need to know to develop your cooking skills. You'll learn about the tools you need and how to use them. You'll learn essential cooking and baking techniques, such as the correct way to chop an onion and how to make whipped cream from scratch. And you'll learn about ingredients and flavors that make recipes taste great.

And as a bonus, you'll get a collection of essential recipes, made with easy-to-find whole foods, that will help you practice the techniques you learn. These recipes were designed for beginners so you can become more comfortable in the kitchen while making delicious food for your family and friends.

How to Use This Book

How to Cook is a reference guide packed with essential information that beginner cooks need to know, and easy and delicious recipes you can easily master. The first two chapters of the book cover kitchen/cooking fundamentals. Chapter 1 focuses on the tools and ingredients you need for a well-stocked kitchen and the skills you will learn to master as you become a more confident cook. Chapter 2 focuses on understanding flavor and the ingredients you'll be cooking with.

Chapters 3 through 8 teach you cooking techniques based on specific types of ingredients. These chapters are broken down by ingredient type and explain how to handle, prep, cook, and store the ingredient. You'll also find easy, flavor-packed recipes that will help you practice the techniques you're learning and start to build a recipe repertoire. Each recipe includes the skills used, such as knife skills and measuring. I've also included shortcuts and troubleshooting tips. Chapter 9 will help you pull together everything you learned. The recipes in this chapter use the various skills you learned in the previous chapters.

The recipes were carefully designed for beginner cooks. They are easy to make and don't require complicated steps or hard-to-find ingredients. But don't feel constrained by these recipes. I encourage you to have the confidence to experiment with flavors, try new things, and make these recipes your own.

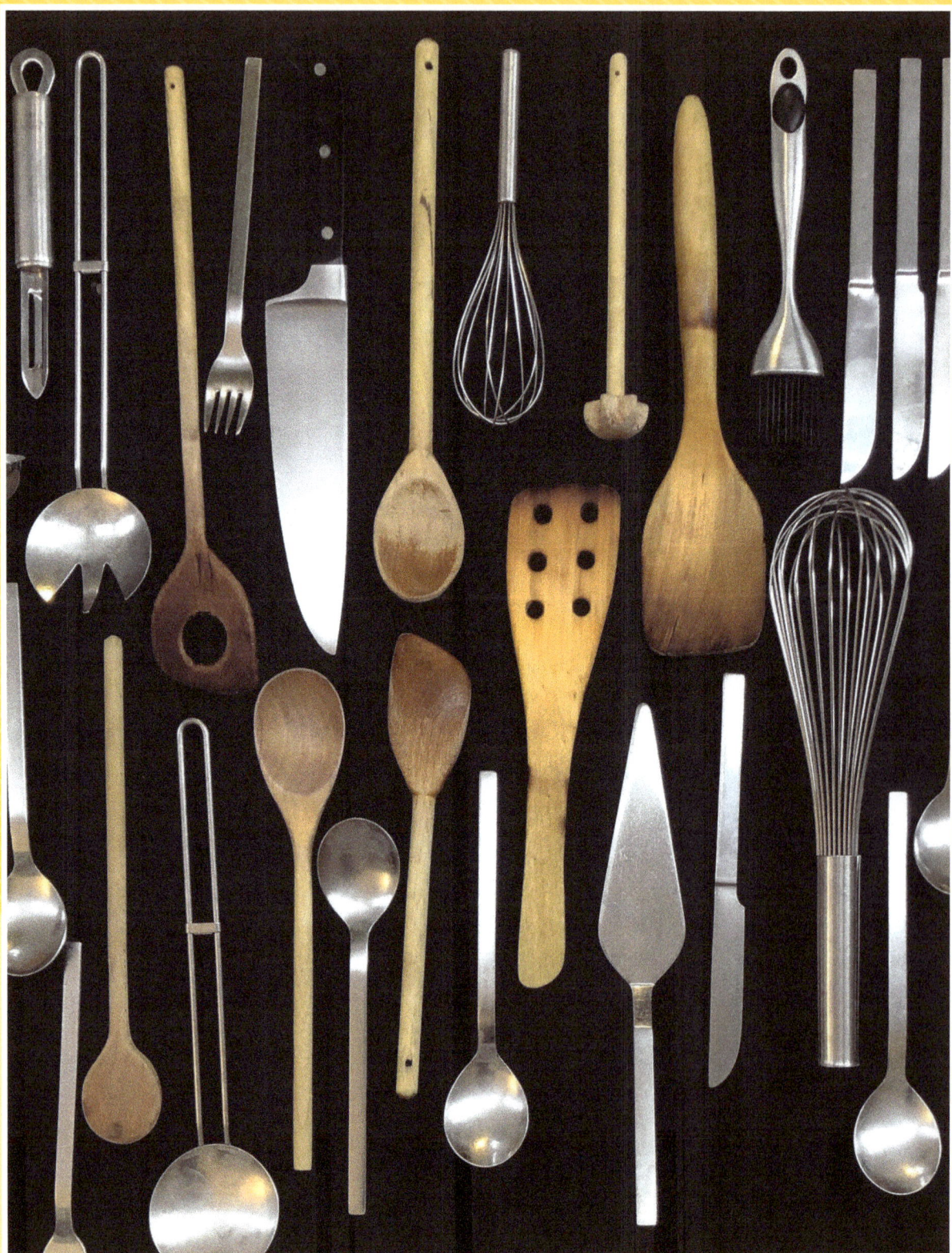

CHAPTER 1

Kitchen Fundamentals

Cooking is much easier when you have everything you need. This chapter will help you get your kitchen (and you) ready to do what it was meant to do . . . cook. It describes the tools, equipment, and skills you need to make the recipes in this book. The chapter also covers some common cooking terms that may or may not already be familiar to you, as well as the safe use of essential cooking gear. And if you've wondered about the difference between chopping and dicing, and don't know whether you should roast or bake, then this chapter is for you.

Welcome to the Kitchen

You've made a smart choice by starting your cooking adventure here. Before you begin cooking, it's important that you have the right tools and ingredients. Setting up your kitchen properly will ultimately set you up for cooking success.

You won't need any complicated gadgets or appliances to make the recipes in this book. You'll be using basic pieces that are the foundation of any well-stocked kitchen. Before you go shopping, though, determine what you already have on hand; you may already have a lot of what you need. You might be surprised by the simplicity of this list of essentials.

Kitchen Essentials

When it comes to cooking and baking, there are some essential tools that you can't do without. For example, a good, sturdy chef's knife that fits well in your hand and a few well-made pots and pans are the workhorses in the kitchen. In the following sections, you'll find recommendations for the types and sizes of what you need. Purchase the best quality that your wallet allows.

BASIC TOOLS

- **Can opener:** A manual or electric can opener is essential for opening canned goods.

- **Colander:** Look for a colander with smaller holes that can drain large items, such as vegetables, and fine items, such as rice.

- **Cutting board:** A solid plastic cutting board is versatile, sturdy, and easy to clean. Look for one that is at least 8 by 10 inches in size. Having more than one helps to prevent cross contamination.

- **Kitchen shears:** These sturdy, heavy-duty scissors are great for all sorts of cooking tasks, including snipping herbs, trimming piecrust, and cutting through hard bones.

Just The Basics Cookbook

- **Knives:** A sharp knife is a cook's best tool. A chef's knife with an 8-inch blade is a great knife for newer cooks. You should also have a paring knife and a serrated knife for cutting bread.

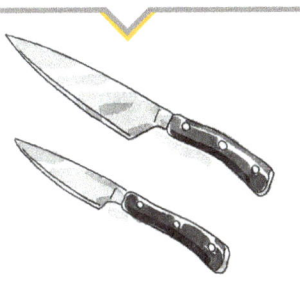

- **Measuring cups and spoons:** You will need three types of measuring tools: a set of dry measuring cups, a liquid measuring cup, and a set of measuring spoons. Learn about the differences in these items in Measure It Out (see page 9).

- **Meat tenderizer:** This gadget is used to tenderize or pound meat into thinner pieces. I recommend a mallet-style with a flat size and a side with triangular teeth.

- **Meat thermometer:** A meat thermometer is the most accurate and efficient way to tell when meat or fish is cooked properly. I recommend a digital thermometer for ease of use.

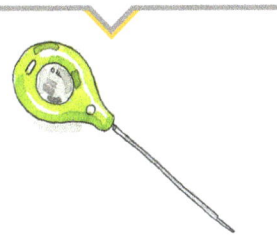

- **Spatulas:** You will need two types of spatulas: a 12-inch silicone scraper spatula for mixing, and a turning spatula for flipping foods.

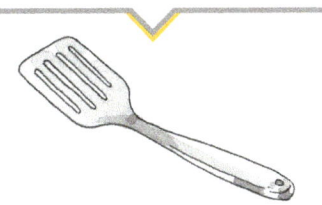

- **Spoons:** It's handy to have a variety of spoons in your kitchen. Spoons with silicone heads are great for mixing and cooking; they won't scratch your pans. You should also have a slotted spoon to drain excess liquid and a ladle for scooping larger portions of liquids.

Kitchen Fundamentals

- **Tongs:** I recommend a sturdy set of 12-inch tongs with silicone tips. These are great for transferring food and for tossing salad.

- **Vegetable peeler:** Choose a comfortable peeler that stays sharp.

- **Whisk:** A whisk is essential when you need to mix ingredients and incorporate some air. Look for an 11- or 12-inch whisk with a comfortable handle.

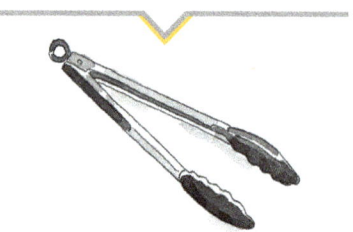

ESSENTIAL COOKING VESSELS

- **Baking dishes:** I recommend having two sizes—a 13-by-9-inch rectangular baking dish and an 8-inch square version. These can be glass or aluminum and are essential for casseroles, cakes, and other baking needs.

- **Dutch oven:** Look for a 4½- to 6-quart Dutch oven with a tight-fitting lid. These pots can be heavy when filled, so comfortable handles are a must.

- **Mixing bowls:** You'll want to have a few mixing bowls on hand, a 3-quart and a 5-quart version. Plastic is fine, but glass is more versatile.

- **Pie dish:** A standard 9-inch pie dish made of either glass or metal is great for making pies and other baked goods.

- **Rimmed baking sheet:** A 15½-by-10-inch aluminum sheet pan with a small rim around the edge is perfect for baking cookies or making sheet pan meals. Larger ones are nice to have as well.

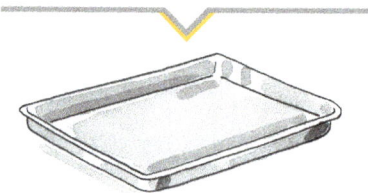

- **Saucepan:** A 3-quart saucepan with a lid is very versatile. This can be used for simmering and boiling.
- **Skillet or frying pan:** A 10-inch skillet or frying pan is a great all-purpose pan. Look for one with a tight-fitting lid. Nonstick or stainless-steel pans are both great options for beginner cooks.

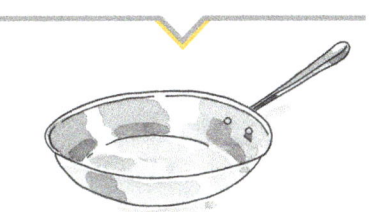

BASIC APPLIANCES

A microwave, food processor, and electric mixer are necessary for the recipes here, but there are other appliances that make your life easier in the kitchen but are not must-haves.

- **Electric hand mixer:** This small appliance makes mixing batters a cinch. Look for a mixer with multiple speeds to prevent splattering.
- **Electric kettle:** This energy-efficent dynamo is excellent for quickly boiling water.
- **Food processor:** Food processors are not only great for pulverizing foods into fine pieces, but they can also be used for mixing and pureeing. Some models even come with blades for shredding, grating, and slicing.
- **Immersion blender:** This no-mess, sticklike blender allows you to blend and puree without taking recipes like soups out of the pot and pouring it into a blender.
- **Knife sharpener:** When knives get dull, they are dangerous. Knives should be sharpened every 1 to 2 months, depending on the amount of use.
- **Microwave:** Microwave power is measured in wattage. Look for a microwave with at least 700 watts.
- **Multi-cooker:** This appliance has many uses—pressure cooking, slow cooking, steaming, braising, and sautéing.
- **Rice Cooker:** This handy appliance is a fuss-free (but not essential) way to make perfect rice every time.

Basic Skills 101

Mastering the basics like reading a recipe, prepping ingredients, and handling a knife will go a long way to making you feel more kitchen efficient and confident as a cook.

MASTER THE KNIFE

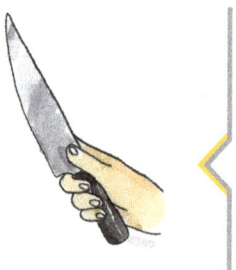

Learning to use a knife properly is one of the most important cooking skills. It may seem intuitive, but it takes some learning. It starts with holding the knife properly. Balance the knife gently in the palm of your hand and wrap your middle, ring, and pinkie fingers around the handle, close to where the handle meets the blade. Place the knuckle of your index finger against the blade on the side of the knife close to the handle, then place your thumb on the opposite side of the blade to grip it firmly.

Use your free hand to hold the food that you're cutting. For safety reasons, curl your fingertips under, resembling a claw, and guide the food toward the blade. Make your cuts in a single motion instead of sawing back and forth. When learning knife skills, focus on precision, not speed.

Below are some basic knife cuts that you'll use:

Chopping: Cutting the item into smaller pieces roughly the same size. When chopping round food items, such as carrots or potatoes, halve them and place the flat side on your cutting surface.

Dicing: Cutting the item into small pieces, about ¾ inch or smaller. Start by slicing the item lengthwise. Then cut the slices lengthwise into thinner pieces. Cut these pieces crosswise into smaller pieces.

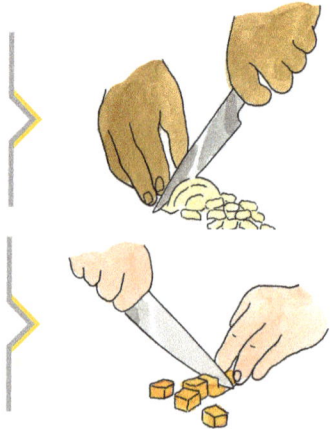

Just The Basics Cookbook

Mincing: Cutting into superfine dice. This technique is usually used with garlic or ginger. Cut the item into thin slices. Keep the tip of the knife blade against the board and place the fingertips of your free hand on top of the blade. Rock the blade back and forth and up and down over the slices, changing direction frequently to cut the item into superfine dice.

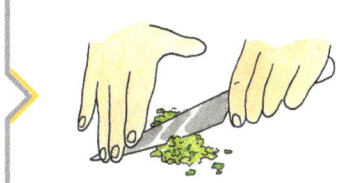

Peeling: Hold the fruit or vegetable firmly in your nondominant hand. Using a peeler, glide the blade across the skin of the produce away from you in steady, even strokes.

Slicing: Cutting the item into broad, thin pieces. Hold the tip of the blade against the board and pull the knife downward in a single motion through the item you are slicing.

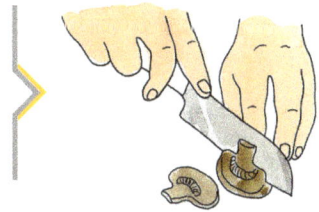

• SAFETY FIRST •

Safety in the kitchen should always be the top priority. From cuts and burns to sickness, there are a number of ways to be injured while cooking. Luckily, most of them are avoidable. Here are some tips to keep you safe:

Always keep a fire extinguisher nearby: Every kitchen should have a fire extinguisher for grease fires. Check your extinguisher periodically to ensure it is properly charged and hasn't expired. You can also snuff out a grease fire by placing a lid or baking sheet on top of the fire or, for small fires, pour salt on it to cover the flames. Never use water on a grease fire.

Avoid cross contamination: Do not reuse a knife or cutting board used to cut raw meat, fish, or seafood. Always wash the utensils and prep area with warm, soapy water after handling these items.

Avoid spoiled food: Make it a habit to regularly go through your refrigerator, freezer, and pantry, and remove expired food and past-their-prime leftovers.

Clean up spills: Spills on the floor can be dangerous in the kitchen. Clean up any spills as soon as they happen.

Cook meats to the proper temperature: The only way to truly know if meat or fish is cooked is a meat thermometer, so I've included proper cooking temperatures in each recipe.

Handle knives with care: Always cut on a clean and stable surface, and if you drop a knife, do not try to catch it. Make sure your knives stay sharp. Dull knives can slip.

Oven safety: Always keep dry potholders or oven mitts nearby and be careful of your arms when reaching in the oven to remove food. It's also important to stand back when opening the oven door.

Prevent burns: Always turn pot handles toward the back of the cooktop so you don't bump them or catch them on your sleeve. Make sure that potholders are dry. Picking up a pot with a damp potholder can cause a burn. Always remove pot lids away from your face to avoid steam burns.

Wash your hands: Before you start cooking, always wash your hands with warm, soapy water. Rewash your hands after handling raw meat or seafood.

MEASURE IT OUT

The success of a recipe, especially baked goods, often depends on precise measurements. When measuring by the teaspoonful or tablespoonful, you should use measuring spoons. Fill the appropriate spoon to the top, and level it off with a straight edge, such as the back of a butter knife.

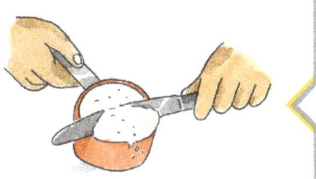

To measure larger portions of dry ingredients, you need a set of dry measuring cups, usually sold in sets ranging from ¼ cup to 1 cup. To properly measure dry ingredients, spoon the ingredient into the appropriate measuring cup. Swipe a straight edge across the top to remove any excess.

To measure wet ingredients, use a transparent measuring cup with graduated measurements and a pouring spout. Place the measuring cup on a level surface and pour the liquid into the cup.

READING A RECIPE

As a new cook, it's important to closely follow a recipe. A well-written recipe will provide everything you need to know to successfully make the dish. It includes the ingredients, instructions, cook time, and number of servings (sometimes referred to as "yield"). Within the instructions, it will tell you the equipment you need, the techniques you will use to cook, and often, how to serve and store the food you've made. Some recipes even include bonus tips, such as more information on an ingredient or how to vary the flavor of a recipe.

When you select a recipe to make, it's important that you carefully read the entire recipe first. You want to make sure you have the correct ingredients and equipment on hand, as well as enough time to make the dish. Be sure to consider any marinating, cooling, or chilling times. I always recommend that you read the recipe twice before starting to cook. Remember, when you're just getting started, the preparation steps might take you a little longer.

The recipe's ingredient list will enumerate the ingredients in the order used in the recipe. Sometimes, ingredients will have a comma with extra notes. When you see this, the instruction after the comma should be completed after the ingredient is measured. For example, "1 cup of fresh parsley leaves, chopped" means you measure out one cup of fresh parsley leaves and then chop them. Conversely, if you see "1 cup chopped fresh parsley leaves," you should chop the parsley leaves before you measure them.

Get Cooking

When learning to cook, it's important to understand the various terminology and techniques. This list describes the basic techniques you will need to make the recipes in this book.

SIMMERING AND BOILING

Simmering and boiling involve cooking liquids on the stove. To simmer, you bring the liquid to just below the boiling point. You will notice small bubbles around the edge of the pot. To boil, bring the liquid to the boiling point. Large bubbles will form and break through the surface of the liquid. Simmering is good for gently cooking stews and sauces, and a vigorous boil is the proper way to cook pasta. Often, a recipe will tell you to bring a liquid to a boil and then reduce it to a simmer, which you can do by simply adjusting the heat.

STEAMING

Steaming involves cooking food by using the steam from a boiling liquid. The food is placed in a vessel on top of the boiling liquid but never touches the liquid. The steam coming off the liquid cooks the food gently. This is a healthy way to prepare food, because most of the nutrients remain and are not cooked off.

GRILLING

Grilling is a form of dry-heat cooking where food is cooked over an open flame or another direct heat source. Grilling can be done using gas, charcoal, or wood and is a quick way to cook food without using much fat, so it's a healthier cooking technique. Grilled food often has a distinct smoky flavor and seared texture.

ROASTING

Roasting is a dry-heat technique that's generally done in an oven. Roasting is done with solid foods, such as meats and vegetables, at higher temperatures (generally 400°F or hotter). This cooking method creates a browned, flavorful coating on the outside of the food.

BAKING

Baking is another form of dry-heat cooking that's done in an oven. Unlike roasting, baking involves foods that don't have much structure until they are cooked, such as a cake. Baking is generally done at a lower temperature, up to 375°F.

SAUTÉING/STIR-FRYING

Sautéing involves heating fat (butter, oil) in a pan and, when hot, adding the food. Once added, you move the food around the pan quickly until it is cooked through. It is important not to overcrowd the pan so that the food can brown and cook evenly. Sautéing is a great way to build flavors in a recipe.

SEARING

Searing involves heating some fat in a pan on a stovetop and lightly frying a protein to develop a crust on the outside. Searing is usually the first step in a cooking process, after which the meat will continue to cook using another cooking method. Searing not only develops flavor, but it also locks in the meat's natural juices.

BRAISING

Braising is a two-step process that involves searing a protein over dry heat, then adding liquid and cooking the meat at a lower temperature until it's cooked through. Braising can be done on a stovetop, in the oven, or in a slow cooker.

BROILING

Broiling uses intense, direct heat from the top of the oven to cook food. Broiling temperatures usually start at 500°F. Broiled foods develop similar char and flavors of grilled foods.

PANFRYING

Panfrying is done on a stovetop and uses oil to cook the food at a constant medium-high temperature. The food has direct contact with the bottom of the pan and develops browning and a crispy texture.

Love Your Oven and Cooktop

The oven is one of the hardest-working appliances in your kitchen. It's great for baking, roasting, braising, and broiling. There are some basic rules you should follow when using this appliance. First, it's important that you maintain consistent heat in the oven. Many recipes instruct you to preheat the oven before cooking. This means before you even start making the recipe, you turn the oven on and let it come up to the desired temperature. It's also important that you don't keep opening the oven door while food is baking or roasting. Every time you open the door, heat will escape, and the oven temperature will lower.

The exception is broiling. Often, the oven temperature will get so hot during the broiling process that the oven will turn off. It helps to keep the oven door cracked a bit to regulate the higher temperature. Be sure to keep a close watch over food under a broiler. It can burn very quickly.

Next, it's important to follow a recipe's baking time. I recommend using a timer. Follow the instructions in the recipe for the cooking times. Start by setting the timer for the shortest time. Check the food and, if it's not quite done, continue to cook it, checking for doneness every few minutes.

It's also critical to follow the recipe's instructions when it comes to rack placement. Some recipes are very specific as to how close to the heat source the food should be placed. You should also note any instructions for rotating baked goods for even baking.

CONVECTION OVEN

Some ovens come equipped with a convection setting. A convection oven has a fan and exhaust system built in that keeps hot air circulating around food as it cooks. Convection cooking allows your food to cook more evenly and quickly than standard ovens. Convection ovens also help with browning. In a standard oven, as food cooks, it gives off moisture that can't escape, creating a humid cooking environment. The fan in a convection oven will move the air around, creating a drier cooking environment, causing food to brown faster.

UNDERSTANDING COOKTOPS

Cooktops or stoves are different than ovens. Sometimes, ovens and cooktops are sold as one unit. The cooktop is on top and the oven is on the bottom. These two appliances can also be separate from each other, with a cooktop on the counter and an oven mounted on the wall.

When it comes to cooktops, there are several types: electric, gas, and induction. Gas cooktops get their heat from a flame. They heat up and cool down quickly. Gas cooktops give you a lot of temperature control. Electric cooktops have coils heated with electricity. They take a little longer to heat up compared to the other types. Induction cooktops use electromagnetism between the pan and the coils to create heat. This keeps the cooktop cool to the touch. The only downside is that you need to make sure your cookware is suited for induction cooking.

Be Prepared

Before you start cooking, it's important that you prep the area. Make ample space to work, and wipe surfaces to prevent any cross contamination. Be sure you have the time you need to complete the recipe. After you've read through the recipe (at least twice), gather the equipment and ingredients. Preheat the oven, if needed.

Next, start prepping the ingredients, such as washing, peeling, and chopping vegetables, grating cheese, measuring ingredients, and opening cans. Prep the meat or seafood last, and keep them refrigerated until you're ready to use them.

The final step is to go through the recipe one more time and double-check that you have everything you need where you want it. At this point, you should be ready to start cooking.

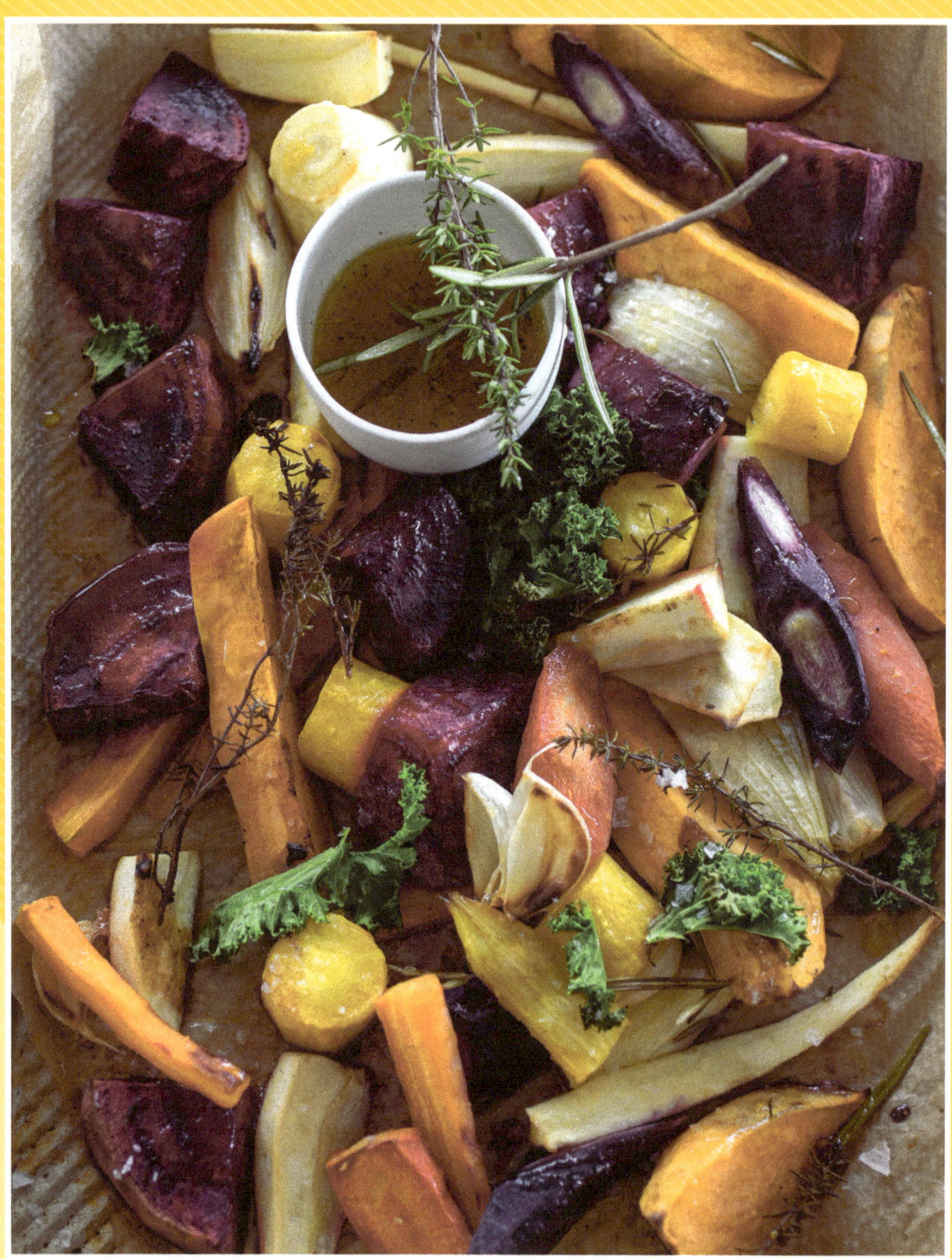
Robust Roasted Root Vegetables, page 53.

CHAPTER 2

How Flavor Develops

How food tastes is actually only one part of flavor. Flavor also involves a number of sensations, including the sense of smell and the feel of the food in our mouths. This chapter delves into what gives our food flavor, what makes it taste great, and why.

Developing Good Flavor

Creating a delicious recipe is an art and a science. What makes food taste good? Understanding the answer to this question is a major component of creating flavorful dishes every time you cook.

Taste is the first thing we think of when it comes to flavor, but several other factors, including aroma, texture, appearance, and temperature, come into play. Our brains process all of these signals and determine if we like something.

Before you even take a bite of food, your eyes tell you if the food looks good, and your nose picks up the aroma. When you take a bite, your mouth feels the texture and temperature of the food, and your taste buds process the flavor. A good recipe will factor in all of these elements.

Five Ways to Taste

The human tongue processes five basic tastes—sweet, salty, sour, bitter, and umami. The best recipes are made up of combinations of these basic tastes. Many recipes stick with common blends like sweet and sour, but sometimes a recipe will push our taste buds outside their comfort zone with something like bacon ice cream.

As a beginner cook, it's helpful to understand the basic tastes and how they work together. This can help you troubleshoot when something goes wrong or make substitutions as you're cooking.

SWEET

The sweet flavor many of us find pleasurable comes from sugar, either natural or processed. Because it's a central energy source, our bodies naturally tend to like it.

SALTY

Salt is a natural flavor enhancer. You'll see it used in many recipes, including cakes and cookies because it helps to balance the sweetness and bring out other flavors. Our taste buds are naturally set to like a little salt flavor. Foods that are naturally salty include tomatoes and anchovies.

SOUR

Sourness tells us that something is acidic. Sourness is primarily found in some fruits and in fermented foods such as vinegar and yogurt. These foods can be intense on their own, but when you use them to enhance recipes, it brings them to life.

BITTER

We are most sensitive to the taste of bitterness. Many toxic elements in nature are bitter. We naturally react when something is bitter because our instincts tell us that bitterness is dangerous. Naturally bitter foods can add interest and flavor to food. Bitter food include coffee, grapefruit, and kale.

UMAMI

Umami is the most newly described of the five flavors. It's described as meaty or savory. Foods like hard cheese, mushrooms, and cured meats are rich in compounds that bring that umami flavor. Cooking foods can also bring out umami flavors. We especially see this when foods brown and flavors intensify.

Building Balanced Flavor and Texture

Now that you understand the basic tastes, you can start to see how combining them produces incredible flavor. Adding texture into the mix will also enhance your understanding of what makes a good recipe and demonstrate how considering one without the other does not work. A good recipe includes contrasting textures, such as crunchy and creamy or soft and crispy.

Building flavor generally requires seasoning food before cooking it or early in the cooking process. Seasoning food will bring out the other flavors and help balance the dish. If you only add salt at the end, for instance, it won't have time to do its job and bring out the natural flavors. It will only make the food taste salty. Another way to build flavor is to add a dash of acidity at the end of cooking. A squeeze of lemon or a splash of vinegar can help cut through heavy flavors and wake up a dish.

Likewise, one of the components of flavor is how food feels in your mouth. This refers to the food's texture. But texture does not only engage the sense of feeling; we also notice it with our eyes. Think about fried chicken. You see the chicken, and without even tasting it, you know it's going to be crispy.

BALANCING THE TASTE PROFILES

Have you ever tasted a dish and thought it was too salty, too sweet, or too bitter? Usually, you can address these problems during the cooking process. When adjusting ingredients in a recipe, you should always start small, adding a little at a time. The more you cook, the better you will become at tasting for flavor and adjusting along the way (except with meat and fish). You will also become more confident in trying new combinations.

When balancing the flavors of a recipe, there are a few guidelines to consider:

Sweet: Balances sourness and bitterness and enhances saltiness

Salty: Balances bitterness and enhances sweetness

Sour: Balances sweetness and bitterness and enhances saltiness

Bitterness: Balances sweetness and saltiness

Umami: Balances bitterness and enhances sweetness

The next time you taste food, stop and think about what tastes you're experiencing, and then consider how you can enhance or balance the flavors you're tasting.

TEXTURE OF THE DISH

When we crave foods, it's not the taste we are craving but the texture. The same is true for foods we don't like. It's often not the taste that we dislike, but how the food feels in our mouths.

Generally, there are five basic textures:

1. Watery, like thinner soups and sauces

2. Firm, like vegetables or chicken

3. Crunchy/crispy, like roasted or fried foods or crackers

4. Creamy, like purees or thicker soups

5. Chewy, like breads, grains, and beans

Food textures can help enhance a recipe and make it more satisfying. For example, consider how croutons or nuts give that salad the crunch it needs, how crusty bread just brings out a bowl of soup, or how tortilla chips are a must-have to dip in guacamole.

Different cooking techniques yield different textures. Grilling, searing, and frying will produce a crisp texture, whereas baking and steaming can yield a chewier texture. All of these factors go into crafting a recipe.

No-Fuss Nutrition

Food is essential, because it provides the vital nutrients your body needs to survive. All food contains macronutrients and micronutrients. Each of these plays a specific role in how the body functions.

Macronutrients include protein, fat, and carbohydrates. Protein—found in meats, fish, seafood, eggs, and legumes—helps build muscle, aids in growth and development, and repairs and maintains the body. Dietary fat—found in oils, milk, meats, and nuts—helps give structure to our cells and helps our bodies absorb certain vitamins. Carbohydrates are the body's main source of energy. Many fruits and vegetables have carbohydrates, as do rice and grains.

Micronutrients are the vitamins and minerals that support overall health. Vitamins help produce energy and aid in healing, immunity, and bone growth. Minerals give structure to our skeletons and support cardiovascular health.

A balanced meal will have all of these components. Foods will often have more than one macro- or micronutrient. For example, legumes (such as lentils or peanuts) have protein, fiber, carbohydrates, and fat. Depending on the type of legume, it may also have various micronutrients. When building a meal, it's important to consider the nutritional value of the various components. A balanced meal should ensure that your body remains full and provide the necessary nutrients.

To compose a balanced meal, incorporate food of various types, such as proteins, fats, carbohydrates, and vegetables, and minimize foods with processed and added sugars. Foods made with whole grains are higher in nutrients than refined versions. Try choosing leaner proteins like fish and using nondairy alternatives, for a heart-healthy diet.

Strive to incorporate colorful food. Generally, the more color a fruit or vegetable has, the better it is for you. When adding fats, look for unsaturated fats, because our bodies need these in moderation. Last, consider portion control. Try to make fruits or vegetables the largest portion of the meal. Be sure to read the food labels to understand the serving size of each item. For more information on portion control, check out the Resources (page 146).

Stock Up on Staples

Flavor also relies upon the ingredients that you use. The recipes in this book use common ingredients you can find in any grocery store. Keeping a well-stocked pantry, refrigerator, and freezer enables you to whip something up last minute. Always check the expiration dates.

PANTRY STAPLES

- **All-purpose flour:** This is the basis for most baked goods and is used as a thickener for sauces. Store flour in an airtight container in a cool, dark place.

- **Sugar:** Granulated and brown sugars can be used in sweet and savory dishes. All types of sugar should be kept in airtight containers at room temperature.

- **Bread:** This is great to have on hand for turning leftovers into sandwiches. Keep soft breads in an airtight bag at room temperature, or freeze sliced bread to defrost as needed.

- **Canned goods:** A variety of canned goods, including vegetables, tomatoes, fish, and beans, are great for simplifying recipes. They have a long shelf life and don't require any special care.

- **Grains:** A variety of rice, oats, quinoa, and other grains can be the foundation for or side dish to many recipes. If you keep grains tightly sealed at room temperature, they should last for quite a while.

- **Oil:** Oils help with browning, not sticking, and they add structure and balance to dressings. The recipes in this book use canola oil and extra-virgin olive oil unless otherwise stated. But feel free to substitute other oils like coconut or avocado. Store oils in a tightly covered container in a cool, dark place.

- **Dried pasta:** Keep a variety of dried pasta shapes on hand for different recipes. Dried pasta should be kept in an airtight container in a cool, dry place.

- **Sauces:** Sauces, such as Worcestershire sauce and soy sauce, can bring great umami flavor to recipes. Read the package for proper storage of individual sauces.

- **Stocks:** Keep a variety of stocks and broths, such as chicken, beef, and vegetable, on hand. These are great for building sauces and soups. Store unopened packages at room temperature and opened containers in the refrigerator.

- **Vinegar:** A variety of vinegars will help add flavor and acidity to recipes. The basics include white vinegar, apple cider vinegar, and balsamic vinegar. These can be stored at room temperature.

FRESH STAPLES

- **Butter:** Butter adds flavor to recipes and helps with browning. The recipes in this book use unsalted butter unless otherwise noted. Store butter in the refrigerator or freezer.

- **Eggs:** Eggs can be prepared on their own or incorporated into other recipes. They provide structure and richness to recipes. Store eggs in the refrigerator.

- **Milk:** Milk adds richness and structure to sauces and soups and adds moisture and fat to baked goods. The recipes in this book use whole milk unless otherwise noted. If you want to substitute other types of milk, you may need to adjust the measurements. Milk should be kept refrigerated; pay attention to expiration dates.

- **Cheese:** Cheese is versatile and adds flavor and texture to dishes. Cheese should be tightly wrapped and stored in the refrigerator. Some of my favorites include Parmesan, cheddar, and Monterey Jack.

- **Fruit:** Keep a variety of fruits on hand for recipes and snacking. Lemons are always good for adding a punch of acidity to recipes. Different types of fruits are stored differently. Pay attention to how the fruit is displayed in the grocery store; if it's in a refrigerated case, it should be kept refrigerated.

- **Vegetables:** It's good to have a variety of vegetables for your recipes. Always keep onions, garlic, and potatoes at the ready. As with fruit, pay attention to how vegetables are stored at the grocery store.

FROZEN STAPLES

Some foods are suitable for freezer storage. Vegetables, fruits, fish, seafood, and nuts are some of the most versatile. Here are some tips to help you get the most out of frozen foods:

- **Wrap or seal food tightly before freezing.** This helps protect the food against freezer burn. You can use foil, plastic wrap, freezer bags, or food storage containers.
- **It's smart to keep your freezer full.** Don't be afraid to stock up when something is on sale. Keeping your freezer full is more efficient, because the cold air has less space to circulate.
- **Freeze food in portions.** If you buy something in bulk or have leftovers, it's best to package the food into portions you can easily thaw and eat.
- **Thaw food properly.** Always thaw food slowly in the refrigerator to prevent bacteria from forming. Make sure you allow enough time for the food to thaw before cooking.
- **Know what to freeze . . .** butter, breads, milk, and stock all freeze perfectly . . .
- **. . . and what not to freeze.** Vegetables with high water content (such as lettuce and cucumbers), egg-based sauces like mayonnaise, cream-based sauces and soups, and fried foods are examples of foods you don't want to freeze. Frozen kale and spinach are available, but the texture, when thawed, is different from their fresh counterparts.

HERBS AND SPICES

Having a collection of basic herbs and spices allows you to give your food a quick flavor boost. Keep herbs and spices in airtight containers at room temperature. Be sure to keep an eye on the expiration dates; they do lose their flavor over time.

- **Cinnamon:** This is most used in baked recipes, but it can also lend a warm flavor to savory dishes.
- **Dried oregano:** This is a fundamental flavoring in many Italian- and Latin-inspired recipes. It's also excellent for adding flavor to most proteins.
- **Garlic powder:** Garlic powder is a versatile seasoning. It's an easy way to add a punch of flavor to many dishes.
- **Ground cumin:** This seasoning is used in Latin, Indian, Middle Eastern, and Asian cuisine. It adds an earthy, aromatic flavor.
- **Onion powder:** Like garlic powder, onion powder is also a great way to add some flavor.
- **Paprika:** Made from ground chili peppers, paprika can add great depth of flavor to recipes. This spice comes in varieties that range from sweet to smoky to hot, so choose one that suits your preferences.
- **Pepper:** Black pepper is a pantry staple. It's best to have a pepper grinder to grind your own black peppercorns, but ground black pepper works just fine.
- **Red pepper flakes:** These give a spicy punch to any recipe, but a little bit goes a long way.
- **Salt:** This is excellent for seasoning food when cooking. Iodized table salt is a great all-purpose variety.
- **Vanilla:** Vanilla extract is used primarily in baking. Not only does it add a deep vanilla flavor, but it also helps enhance other flavors. Choose pure vanilla extract over imitation vanilla.

• SHOP RIGHT •

Going to the grocery store can be daunting for new cooks. Use these tips to get the most out of your shopping experience.

1. **Be prepared.** Plan out your menus, read your recipes, scour the sale circulars, and create a shopping list before heading to the market. When you're cooking and run out of an ingredient, immediately add it to an ongoing shopping list.

2. **Understand the layout.** Grocery stores display fresh foods, such as fruits, vegetables, meats, and dairy, in the outer aisles. Pantry staples can be found in the center aisles.

3. **Choose produce wisely.** Produce that is in season will be front and center. It's usually more flavorful and affordable. Don't be afraid to pick up produce to see how it feels. Generally, fresh produce has smooth, unwrinkled skin and feels heavy for its size.

4. **Avoid food waste.** When shopping, stick to your list and don't shop on an empty stomach. If you need to stock up on something, plan to freeze it as soon as you get home.

5. **Buy smaller portions.** If you're cooking for one or two people, you don't have to purchase big packages of food. You can ask the store butcher to cut smaller portions of meats. If the store has a salad bar, it's a great way to purchase single servings of fruits and vegetables.

About the Recipes

In the following chapters, you will learn about cooking different foods. Each chapter covers specific cooking methods and provides tips for making the most of each ingredient. After that, there are featured recipes to get your hands dirty, literally, and allow you to practice the skills you're learning.

TIPS AND TECHNIQUES

Each recipe in this book includes a tip to help you make the most of the recipe and develop your cooking chops further. These tips include:

- **Flavor Boost:** Suggestions for adding ingredients to enhance a recipe's flavor.
- **Ingredient:** Tips for selecting the best ingredient and working with it.
- **Substitution:** Suggestions for swapping out an ingredient to make it leaner, dairy-free, nut-free, grain-free, vegetarian, or vegan.
- **Variation:** Ideas for optional ingredients you can incorporate to change up the recipe.
- **Troubleshooting:** Advice for fixing common cooking errors.
- **General:** Extra instructions to help you successfully cook the dish.

    Now it's time to put this new knowledge to work, and jump right in.

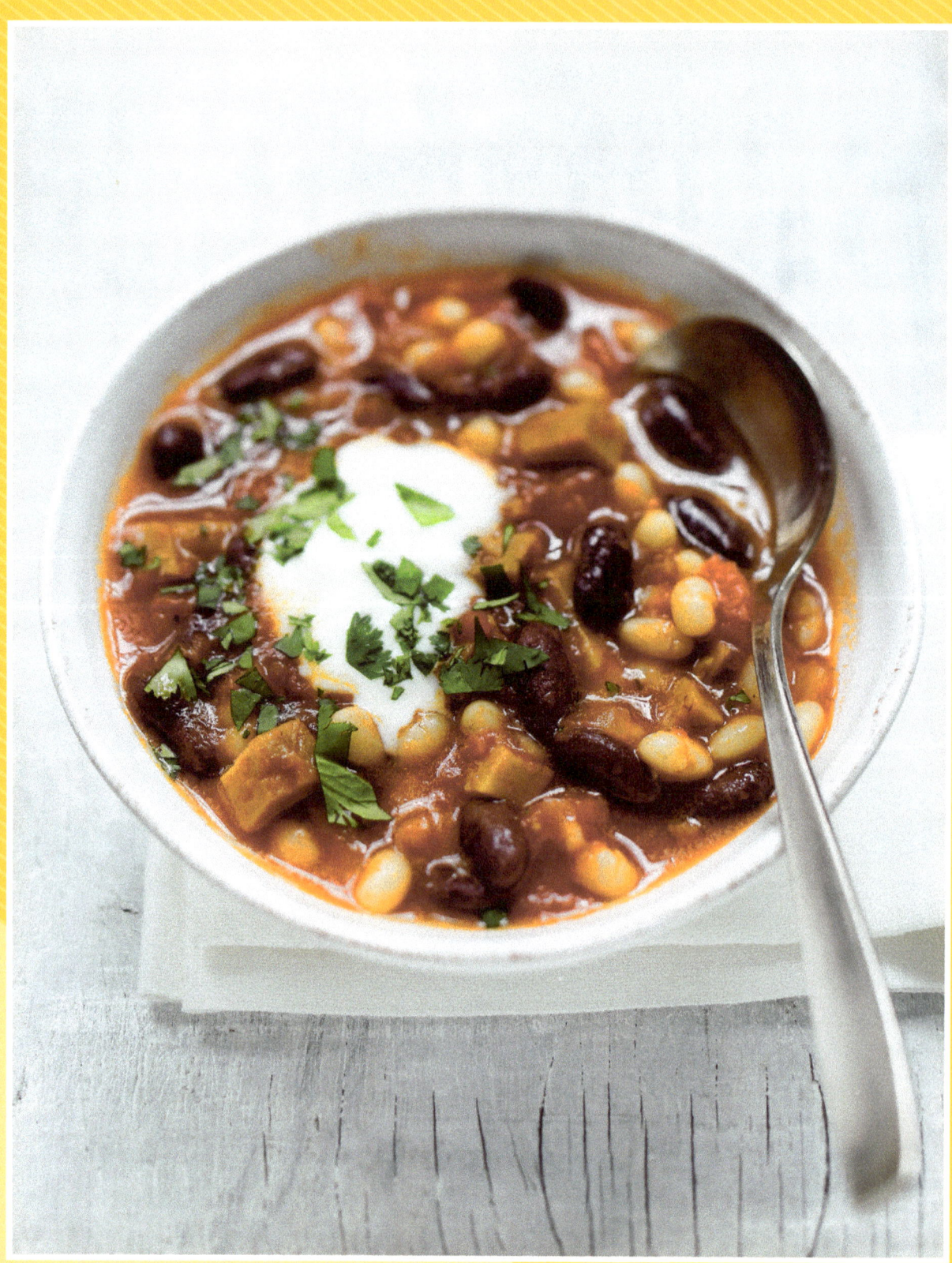
No-Sweat Three-Bean Chili, page 34.

CHAPTER 3

Beans, Grains, and Pastas

Beans, grains, and pastas are great additions to healthy, well-balanced meals; they offer proteins, carbohydrates, and various vitamins and minerals. Most starches have mild flavors, allowing them to absorb the flavors they're cooked with. All of them are a great addition to your cooking repertoire in different ways. Some specific methods and tips will help you prepare beans, grains, and pastas like a pro.

No-Sweat Three-Bean Chili 34

Creamy Risotto 36

Simple Rice Pilaf 38

Velvety Pasta Carbonara 40

Veggie Ramen Bowl 42

With the Grain

Wheat, rice, oats, cornmeal, quinoa, and barley are all grains. Typically, you'll see grains classified as "whole grains" or "refined grains." Whole grains, which include the entire kernel, are the healthier option. Refined grains are processed, and the outer kernel is removed. This gives the grain a finer texture, but it removes many of the nutrients. To add more whole grains to your diet, choose foods labeled as "whole grain," "whole wheat," or "stone-ground whole grain." Brown rice, oats, and wheatberries are examples of whole grains. Most of these whole grains have a cooking process similar to rice. You simply put the grain in a pan with water or another liquid, such as broth or stock, and bring it to a boil. Once it reaches a boil, turn the heat down so the liquid simmers, and cook until the grain absorbs the liquid.

RICE

Rice is the edible seed of a grass and is widely used in many cuisines throughout the world, from risotto and jambalaya to sushi and paella. Rice comes in long, medium, and short grains. Within these varieties, there are many types, textures, and flavors. Some of the common rice varieties include long-grain white rice, brown rice, black rice, basmati rice, jasmine rice, arborio rice, sticky rice, and sushi rice.

Rice is extremely popular because it's plentiful, inexpensive, textural, and filling. It's also a great way to add more substance to a dish or stretch a recipe to feed more people. Rice of any type is very easy to prepare. Check the product package for rice-to-water ratios and cooking times and see How to Cook Rice (page 31).

Noodles and Pasta

People often use the terms "noodles" and "pasta" interchangeably; however, they are different. Noodles are typically made of softer wheat (or other grains, such as rice) and include salt to develop a softer dough. On the other hand, pasta is made with harder wheat, with no salt in the dough. Noodles are often used in recipes from Asia, whereas pasta is used in European recipes.

Very broadly speaking, noodles are consistent in size, but pasta can come in various sizes, shapes, and types. You'll find short types, such as elbows and orzo; long types, such as spaghetti and fettuccini, sheet pasta, such as lasagna; stuffed pasta, such as ravioli; and dumplings, such as gnocchi. The shape and size of pasta you use depends on what you're making. Long, thinner pasta is great for lighter, smoother sauces, whereas shorter pasta is perfect for heartier, chunkier sauces. You'll also find several types of pasta, such as classic or refined, whole wheat, and even chickpea.

All types of noodles and pasta are cooked in salted, boiling water. The amount of time depends on the type and thickness, so you should check the package directions. See How to Cook Pasta (page 30).

Beans and Legumes

Beans and legumes are fiber- and protein-filled powerhouses that also contain many of the vitamins and minerals your body needs to thrive. There are many different varieties of legumes; the types you may be familiar with include dried and fresh beans, soybeans, lentils, chickpeas, peas, and peanuts. Some of the most common beans are kidney, lima, black, great northern, cannellini, and pinto beans.

Most legumes and beans are sold dried or canned, but some can be purchased frozen, such as peas and edamame. Which one you choose depends on cost, taste, and convenience. Canned beans and legumes are much more convenient to prepare (simply open the can and use them), but the trade-off is more cost and less taste. Dried beans and legumes are extremely inexpensive compared to their canned counterparts, and the flavor and texture are far superior; you can control how they are seasoned. If you want to prepare dried beans and legumes, it does entail a few extra steps and a little more time. See How to Soak and Cook Beans (page 32).

Prepping Rice, Pasta, Noodles, Beans, and Legumes

When cooking with rice, dry beans, and legumes, first check for impurities like deformed beans or stones, then rinse them in a strainer under cool water. Pasta and noodles do not require this type of examination.

Most beans, legumes, grains, and pastas are cooked in boiling or simmering salted liquid. The exception is canned beans or legumes. Drain and rinse these items before using them to remove any excess salt from the canning process. Canned beans and legumes are precooked before the canning process, so you can simply heat them through or just enjoy them cold.

How to Cook Pasta

Pasta should be cooked in heavily salted boiling water. You can use any size pot as long as it's large enough to fully submerge the pasta as soon as it's added to the water and it has room to move around as it boils.

BEST PRACTICES

First, bring the water to a boil, then add the salt and the dried pasta. Always stir the pasta after adding it to the boiling water to prevent it from sticking together. Allow the pasta to boil, uncovered, for the instructed time (check the package instructions). It's important to note that fresh pasta will take much less cooking time than dried pasta. Pasta is done cooking when it's "al dente," which means it has a slight firmness in the center. When the pasta is finished cooking, carefully pour the pasta and water into a strainer set in a clean sink. Now it's ready to go.

A couple of things to keep in mind when cooking pasta. The water must come to a complete boil before adding the pasta. This allows the pasta's surface to cook quicker so the interior of the pasta has time to hydrate thoroughly. It's also important that you adequately salt the cooking water. A good rule of thumb is to use 1 tablespoon of salt for 4 quarts of cooking liquid and 1 pound of dried pasta.

TROUBLESHOOTING MISTAKES

When it comes to cooking pasta, there are two common mistakes: undercooking and overcooking. The best way to avoid either extreme is to test pasta a minute before the package instructions say it will be done. Carefully remove a piece of pasta from the cooking water and bite into it. It should be slightly firm and not gummy.

If, however, you drain the pasta and determine that it's undercooked, there is an easy fix: Simply bring more water to a full boil, and add the undercooked pasta. Allow it to cook for another minute or so until it's ready.

If the pasta is overcooked, it will have a gummy or mushy texture. When this happens, the best fix is to sauté it in a bit of olive oil over medium-high heat. Cook it until it firms up a bit but doesn't brown.

How to Cook Rice

Cooking perfect, fluffy rice requires a few simple steps. This basic technique can be used for most types of rice and many other grains, as well. The first step is to measure the dry rice and place it into a strainer. Rinse the rice under cool water until the water runs clear. This removes the excess starch from the outside of the kernel and will prevent the rice from becoming gummy.

BEST PRACTICES

Place the rinsed rice into the pot and add the required water and salt. It's important to start the rice with cold water so the grains cook evenly. Bring the rice to a boil, give it a quick stir, cover the pot, and reduce the heat to low. Once you put the lid on the pot, do not remove it, because rice relies on the steam from the simmering liquid to cook it through. The cooking time will depend on the type of rice; it can range from about 15 minutes for white rice to 45 minutes for brown rice. Be sure to check the package instructions.

When the rice has finished cooking, turn off the heat, and allow the pot to sit, covered, for a few minutes to absorb the last bit of liquid. After a few minutes, remove the lid, and use a fork to fluff the rice, allowing the remaining steam to escape.

Beans, Grains, and Pastas

One of my favorite ways to boost the flavor of rice is to cook it in stock or broth instead of water. If you use unsalted or low-salt broth or stock, you will still need to add salt when cooking. If you find yourself making a lot of rice, investing in a rice cooker might make sense.

TROUBLESHOOTING MISTAKES

Like pasta, the most common mistakes when cooking rice are overcooking and undercooking it. If the rice is crunchy or has a hard texture, you've most likely undercooked it. To fix the problem, add up to ½ cup of water to a pot with the overcooked rice, and put the lid on. Bring the liquid to a simmer, and cook it for a few more minutes.

If the rice is cooked to your liking, but there is still water left in the pot, simply strain it like pasta. But if the rice is overcooked and mushy, there isn't much you can do except turn it into rice pudding. Add equal parts of cooked, plain rice and milk to a saucepan. Bring the mixture to a boil, reduce the heat, and simmer for 15 minutes. The mixture should have a pudding-like texture. Add sugar and vanilla to taste, and enjoy.

How to Soak and Cook Beans

Soaking dried beans is essential to speed up the cooking process. There are two common methods for soaking beans—the overnight method and the quick soak method. Both methods are quite simple and equally effective. For both methods, you will first need to rinse the beans in a strainer and inspect for any debris or imperfect beans.

BEST PRACTICES

For an overnight soak, transfer the rinsed beans to a pot large enough to hold the beans and enough water to cover them by two inches. Add 1 tablespoon of salt per pound of beans, cover the pot, and allow it to sit at room temperature overnight.

For the quick soak method, place the rinsed beans in a pot large enough to hold beans and enough water just to cover them. Add 1 tablespoon of salt per pound of beans. Bring the beans to a boil, turn off the heat, and place a lid on the pot. Let the beans sit for between 1 and 4 hours. Now the beans are ready to be cooked.

The most important thing to remember when soaking beans is to use a large enough pot. The beans will expand in volume as they soak. Add aromatics such as herbs or garlic to make the beans even more flavorful during the cooking process.

TROUBLESHOOTING MISTAKES

When it comes to soaking and cooking beans, the most common mistake is using old beans. Out-of-date dried beans will not soften as easily or at all. Always check the freshness date on the package before cooking. Beans will lose vitamins after two to three years, and the flavor will begin changing after 5 years. If the beans are fresh yet still not softening, it can be due to hard or chlorinated tap water. Try using bottled water when soaking and cooking beans. Acid can also affect the softness of beans, so add acidic ingredients such as vinegar, citrus, tomatoes, or onions *after* the beans are tender.

No-Sweat Three-Bean Chili

Serves 4	**Prep time:** 10 minutes, plus overnight to soak	**Cook time:** 1 hour 15 minutes

Skills used: Dicing, measuring, soaking beans

- ⅓ cup dried black beans, soaked overnight
- ⅓ cup dried kidney beans, soaked overnight
- ⅓ cup dried pinto beans, soaked overnight
- 1¾ teaspoons table salt, divided
- 1 tablespoon canola oil
- 1 cup diced yellow onion (from 1 medium onion)
- 1 cup diced red bell pepper (from 1 medium pepper)
- 1 tablespoon chili seasoning mix
- 1 (28-ounce) can crushed tomatoes
- 2 cups low-sodium vegetable broth
- ¼ teaspoon freshly ground black pepper

Per Serving: Calories: 257; Fat: 5g; Saturated fat: 0g; Cholesterol: 0mg; Carbohydrates: 43g; Fiber: 13g; Protein: 13g; Sodium: 1,332mg

This hearty dish is filled with protein and fiber-rich beans, along with enough seasonings and veggies to make this vegetarian chili the star of any tailgate. You'll get to try out soaking dried beans here, but if you don't have the time, canned beans (see Ingredient Tip) will work. Bonus: The flavor of this chili gets better the longer it sits, which makes it a great make-ahead meal. Use leftovers on top of nachos with some Classic Guacamole (page 130) or spoon it on top of a burger to make a chili burger.

1. Drain the soaked beans and put them in a large pot. Add enough water to cover the beans by 2 inches. Put a lid on the pot, and bring it to a boil over medium-high heat. Reduce the heat to bring the beans to a simmer.

2. After 30 minutes, add 1 teaspoon salt. Continue to simmer for another 30 minutes. Periodically, check the water level to make sure it hasn't evaporated. The beans are done when they are tender. Drain the cooking water, and set them aside.

3. While the beans are cooking, in a large Dutch oven, heat the canola oil over medium-high heat. Add the onion and bell pepper, and cook, stirring occasionally until soft, 5 to 7 minutes. Add the chili seasoning, and stir until fragrant, 1 to 2 minutes.

4. Stir in the crushed tomatoes, vegetable broth, cooked beans, ¾ teaspoon salt, and the black pepper until combined. Bring it to a simmer, and cook for 15 minutes, stirring occasionally until the chili has thickened slightly. Serve warm.

5. To store the leftovers, cool the chili completely, place it in a container with a tight-fitting lid, and refrigerate for up to 4 days.

INGREDIENT TIP: Make this recipe even simpler by substituting canned beans for the dried beans. Use 1 (15-ounce) can of each type of bean. Drain and rinse the beans before adding them in step 3.

Creamy Risotto

| Serves 4 | **Prep time:** 10 minutes | **Cook time:** 30 minutes |

Skills used: Mincing, measuring, sautéing

- 5 cups low-sodium chicken stock or broth
- 2 tablespoons extra-virgin olive oil
- 3 tablespoons unsalted butter, divided
- 1 medium shallot, finely minced
- 3 garlic cloves, finely minced
- 2 cups arborio rice
- 1 cup dry white wine
- ¼ cup grated Parmesan cheese
- ¼ cup heavy (whipping) cream
- Table salt
- ¼ teaspoon freshly ground black pepper

Per Serving: Calories: 638; Fat: 24g; Saturated fat: 11g; Cholesterol: 49mg; Carbohydrates: 82g; Fiber: 3g; Protein: 12g; Sodium: 223mg

Risotto is a great comfort food on a crisp fall night. It is made from arborio rice, which hails from Italy and is creamier and chewier than other short-grain rice. It isn't difficult to make, but you do need to be patient and stir continually. Serve it as a side dish, or if you want to make it a meal, add cooked Italian sausage or shrimp and steamed peas.

1. In a medium saucepan, bring the chicken stock to a light simmer over medium-low heat.

2. In another large pot, heat the olive oil and 2 tablespoons of the butter over medium heat until the butter is melted. Add the shallot and garlic to the butter mixture, and cook until tender, being careful not to brown the shallot or garlic, about 4 minutes. Add the arborio rice, and stir for 2 minutes, making sure the rice is evenly coated with the butter mixture.

3. Add the white wine, and stir until the wine is completely absorbed by the rice, about 3 minutes. Add one cup of the hot stock, and stir until the rice has absorbed all of it. Continue adding stock, 1 cup at a time, stirring until it is absorbed, about 18 minutes total.

4. Test the rice for doneness. The rice kernels should be perfectly al dente, and the sauce should be creamy without being runny. If not, return to the heat, and stir. Taste the rice for doneness every minute until al dente.

5. Remove the rice from the heat, and stir in the grated Parmesan cheese and remaining 1 tablespoon butter. When the butter has melted, stir in the heavy cream. Taste the risotto; add salt to taste and add the pepper. Serve warm.

6. To store leftovers, allow the risotto to cool completely, place it in a container with a tight-fitting lid, and refrigerate for up to 4 days.

TROUBLESHOOTING TIP: Risotto requires continual stirring. Don't walk away or get distracted, because it can stick and burn very quickly.

Simple Rice Pilaf

Serves 4	**Prep time:** 15 minutes	**Cook time:** 35 minutes

Skills used: Dicing, shredding, mincing, measuring, sautéing, cooking rice

¾ cup basmati rice
2 tablespoons unsalted butter
⅓ cup finely diced yellow onion
1 garlic clove, minced
2 cups low-sodium chicken broth
¼ cup dry white wine (see both Tips)
2 tablespoons shredded carrot
2 tablespoons finely diced red bell pepper
1 teaspoon table salt
¼ teaspoon freshly ground black pepper
2 tablespoons slivered almonds
1 tablespoon minced fresh parsley

Per Serving: Calories: 224; Fat: 8g; Saturated fat: 4g; Cholesterol: 15mg; Carbohydrates: 32g; Fiber: 1g; Protein: 4g; Sodium: 587mg

Rice pilaf elevates standard cooked rice because it's toasted and coated in aromatics before it's even cooked. This recipe gets its great texture, color, and flavor from the vegetables and almonds. Pair it with Lemon Butter Fish Packets (page 68) for a hard-to-beat meal.

1. Rinse the rice in a strainer under cool water until the water runs clean. Drain well.

2. In a medium saucepan, melt the butter over medium heat. Once the butter has melted, add the onion, and cook until softened, 3 to 5 minutes. Stir in the garlic, and cook for 1 minute. Add the rice, and stir until it's coated in the butter mixture and starts to toast, 7 to 9 minutes.

3. Now add the chicken broth, white wine, carrot, bell pepper, salt, and black pepper. Raise the heat to bring it to a boil, cover, and reduce heat to simmer. Simmer for 15 to 20 minutes or until the rice absorbs all the liquid.

4. While the rice is simmering, in a dry skillet, toast the slivered almonds over medium heat. Stir occasionally, and allow the nuts to toast for 4 to 5 minutes or until golden brown. Remove them from the heat and set aside.

5. When the rice is finished, turn off the heat and let it sit, covered, for 5 minutes. Remove the lid, fluff with a fork, and stir in the toasted almonds and minced parsley.

6. To store leftovers, allow the dish to cool completely, place it in a container with a tight-fitting lid, and refrigerate for up to 4 days.

INGREDIENT TIP: Choose a wine that you enjoy. When cooking with wine, the liquid reduces, and the flavor intensifies. Dry white wines that work well include pinot grigio, sauvignon blanc, or an unoaked chardonnay.

SUBSTITUTION TIP: If you don't have wine or prefer not to use it, you can substitute equal amounts of water or additional chicken broth.

Velvety Pasta Carbonara

| Serves 6 | **Prep time:** 10 minutes | **Cook time:** 15 minutes |

Skills used: Mincing, chopping, whisking, cooking pasta

1 pound spaghetti
1 tablespoon table salt, plus more for seasoning
1 tablespoon extra-virgin olive oil
8 bacon slices, chopped
2 garlic cloves, minced
3 large eggs
1 cup grated Parmesan cheese, divided
¼ teaspoon freshly ground black pepper

Per Serving: Calories: 479; Fat: 16g; Saturated fat: 6g; Cholesterol: 123mg; Carbohydrates: 59g; Fiber: 2g; Protein: 23g; Sodium: 696mg

Carbonara is one of the four classic Roman pastas. And for good reason; it is a creamy pasta dish made with eggs, cheese, and, classically, guanciale (pork jowl), though here we use bacon. It's just perfect for nights when you're tired but craving a satisfying meal. You can punch the flavor up by adding a squeeze of lemon juice at the end.

1. Bring a large pot of water to a boil. When the pasta water is boiling, add the spaghetti and 1 tablespoon of salt. Make sure the spaghetti is fully submerged, and cook according to the package directions, which will vary with the type of spaghetti (white, wheat, etc.) you're using.

2. While the pasta is cooking, in a large skillet, heat the olive oil over medium-high heat. Add the chopped bacon, and cook until crispy, 5 to 7 minutes. Remove the bacon pieces from the skillet, leaving the bacon fat, and transfer them to a paper-towel-lined plate. Cook the garlic in the same skillet with the bacon fat for 30 seconds over medium heat. Transfer the cooked garlic to a large bowl.

3. In a medium bowl, combine the eggs and ½ cup of the grated Parmesan cheese. Whisk until they are fully combined.

4. When the pasta is done cooking, carefully remove 1 cup of the pasta water and set aside. Using tongs, transfer the cooked spaghetti to the large bowl with the garlic, and add the bacon to the bowl.

5. Working quickly, while the spaghetti is hot, pour in the egg mixture and toss to combine with the tongs. If the mixture seems dry, slowly add some of the reserved pasta water until it's creamy, and the pasta is coated evenly in the sauce.

6. Toss in and combine the remaining grated Parmesan cheese. Taste for seasoning, and add more salt to taste and the black pepper.

7. To store leftovers, allow the dish to cool completely, place it in a container with a tight-fitting lid, and refrigerate for up to 3 days.

TROUBLESHOOTING TIP: If the finished dish seems too goopy or wet, add extra grated Parmesan cheese, ⅛ cup at a time, until you get the desired consistency. If the finished dish is too dry, slowly add more reserved pasta water until you achieve the desired consistency.

SUBSTITUTION TIP: Use turkey bacon instead for a leaner choice.

Veggie Ramen Bowl

Serves 2	**Prep time:** 5 minutes	**Cook time:** 20 minutes

Skills used: Knife skills, measuring, sautéing, cooking noodles

1 teaspoon sesame oil
1 teaspoon canola oil
½ cup shredded carrots
½ cup shiitake mushrooms, stemmed and sliced
2 garlic cloves, minced
2 teaspoons peeled and freshly grated ginger (from a ½-inch piece)
4 cups low-sodium chicken broth
3 tablespoons reduced-sodium soy sauce
1 tablespoon rice vinegar
2 (3-ounce) packages ramen
1 scallion, green parts only, sliced
2 teaspoons sriracha (optional)

Per Serving: Calories: 433; Fat: 19g; Saturated fat: 7g; Cholesterol: 0mg; Carbohydrates: 55g; Fiber: 4g; Protein: 11g; Sodium: 1,929mg

Take ramen beyond the dorm room walls, and create an easy, satisfying dinner that will make the weekly rotation. This cost-effective recipe gives you ample opportunity to practice your knife skills. Plus, you can add your own flair with any toppings that you want, such as shredded chicken or pork, a soft-boiled egg, toasted sesame seeds, chopped cilantro, or just a simple squeeze of lime juice.

1. In a large saucepan, heat the sesame oil and canola oil over medium heat. Add the carrots and mushrooms, and sauté until softened, 1 to 2 minutes, stirring frequently. Add the garlic and ginger, and stir until fragrant, about 30 seconds.

2. Pour in the chicken broth, soy sauce, and rice vinegar, and bring to a simmer. Simmer for 5 minutes. Add the ramen (discard the flavor packets) to the saucepan, and cook according to the package directions, 4 to 6 minutes.

3. When the noodles are cooked through, transfer the dish to serving bowls, and divide the sliced scallions evenly over each bowl. Add sriracha (if using).

4. To store leftovers, allow the ramen to cool completely. Remove the noodles from the broth, and store the broth and noodles in separate containers with tight-fitting lids. Refrigerate for up to 4 days.

SUBSTITUTION TIP: Make this a vegetarian dish by replacing the chicken stock with vegetable stock.

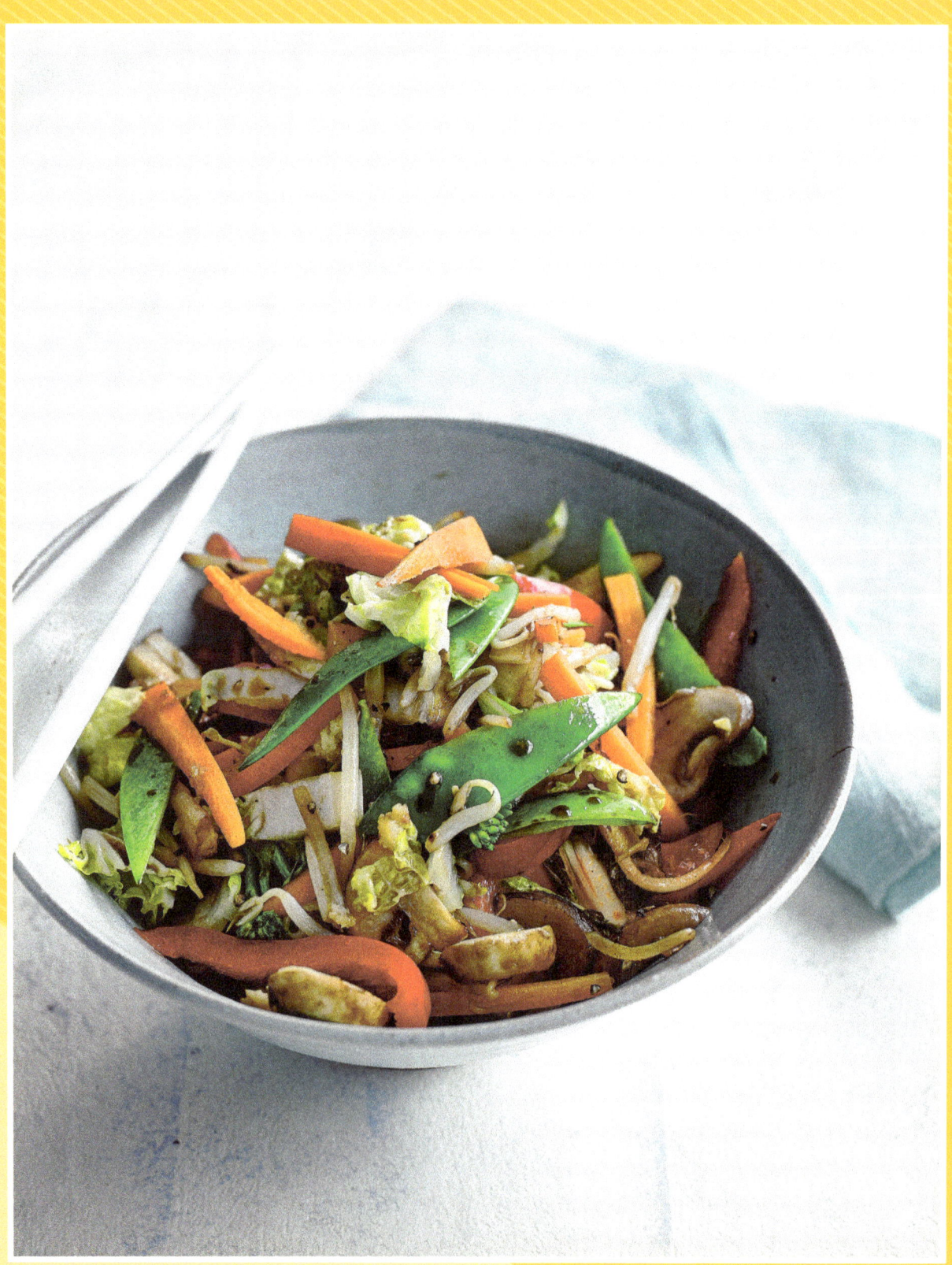

Rainbow Stir-Fry, page 54.

CHAPTER 4

Fruits and Vegetables

Fruits and vegetables provide us with many of the vitamins and nutrients that our bodies need. And they cover the cuisine gamut from salads to apple pies. Try to incorporate a wide variety of colors when selecting fruits and vegetables for your diet.

Classic Tossed Salad with Homemade Vinaigrette 51

Mashed Potatoes in a Snap 52

Robust Roasted Root Vegetables 53

Rainbow Stir-Fry 54

Easy as Apple Crisp 55

Fruity Flavor

Fruit is the edible, sweet, and fleshy product of a tree or plant usually containing seeds. There are several common types of fruit: Apples and pears, citrus, stone fruit, tropical fruit, melons, berries, and tomatoes and avocados (yup, these are fruit). If you want the freshest and sweetest fruit, it's best to purchase it directly from the grower; check out your local farmers' market or farm stand. Grocery stores carry an abundance of all types of fresh fruit, making them quick, easy, and convenient. Many grocers will also carry fruit from local growers.

When selecting the best fruit, use your senses. Look at it. Feel it. Smell it. It is easy to tell if certain fruits—such as berries and apples—are fresh just by looking at them. These fruits should be brightly colored and without blemishes. Melons and tropical fruits can be trickier. Look for glossy, bright fruit. Feel, don't squeeze, for tenderness; there should be a slight give without being too hard or mushy. Does the fruit smell like it should? Peaches should smell peachy. There are some common signs that fruit is beyond its peak freshness. Look for dark spots or bruising on the exterior of the fruit. Fruit beyond its prime may also look shriveled or dried out.

You may be wondering if purchasing organic produce is better. Organic produce has lower levels of pesticides than conventional produce, but the nutritional value is pretty consistent between the two.

WHAT'S IN SEASON

Fruit is more plentiful and less expensive when in season and locally sourced, as are vegetables. Items such as berries and stone fruits are fresher, sweeter, and less expensive when they are in season locally. Or, if you live in a warmer climate, you can often find tropical fruits and melons at lower prices than in northern climates. Other fruits, such as bananas, citrus, pears, and apples, are widely available and affordable all year long. If you're not sure what's in season in your area, a good rule of thumb is to see what fruits are displayed in the front of the produce section.

Veg Out

Vegetables are typically classified according to the part of a plant that is eaten. The most common varieties include leafy greens, such as lettuce or spinach; root vegetables, such as potatoes and yams; cruciferous veggies, such as broccoli and cabbage; marrow vegetables, such as pumpkins and cucumbers; edible plant stems, such as celery and asparagus; and alliums, such as onions and garlic.

The best way to cook vegetables depends on the type. Harder vegetables, such as carrots and potatoes, can withstand higher cooking temperatures. More tender vegetables, such as spinach, are better when cooked at lower temperatures. Vegetables made of a lot of water, such as cucumbers or lettuce, are best eaten raw.

When selecting vegetables, consider the color and firmness. Look for vegetables that feel firm or crisp to the touch and don't have any soft spots. Inspect the color. Look for bright colors, and watch out for yellowing or browning; this can signal that a vegetable is past its prime. If you buy canned vegetables, avoid dented, leaking, or bulging cans.

CANNED AND FROZEN PRODUCE

In some cases, canned or frozen varieties are great alternatives to fresh. They often contain the same nutritional value. Often, these items are picked and processed at the peak of freshness, providing a convenient and affordable alternative to fresh produce, especially when the produce isn't in season. It's important to note the freshness date on the package.

When working with frozen produce, you may need to thaw the vegetables before incorporating them into your recipes. In this case, make sure you drain the vegetables before adding them. When cooking with canned vegetables, drain and discard the canning liquid (unless the recipe instructs otherwise).

Prepping Fruits and Vegetables

Thoroughly clean vegetables before cooking or eating because they travel a while to get to you, have been handled by others, and may contain pesticides. It's best to clean produce right before using it, because added moisture can speed up decay. The best way to clean produce is to wash it with cool water, then thoroughly dry it. The exception to this is mushrooms. Place mushrooms in a bowl with cool water, and agitate them a bit, allowing the dirt to settle to the bottom of the bowl. Remove the mushrooms, and pat them dry.

When storing fresh vegetables, leave them attached to their stems to keep them from drying out. When you are ready to use the vegetable, peel it and cut it.

Most refrigerators come with a produce drawer designed to maintain the proper humidity level for storing produce. If you're storing leftover produce that has been cut, place it in an airtight container or bag, and store it in the refrigerator. Use it within 1 to 2 days.

How to Core an Apple

Removing the core from an apple is simpler than it seems and involves just a chef's knife and a cutting board.

BEST PRACTICES

If you want to peel the apple, do so before coring. Then place the apple upright on a cutting board. Use the chef's knife to cut the apple in half from top to bottom. Place the cut sides down on the cutting board. Cut each half in half again. Place each quarter with a flat side down on the cutting board. Cut into each quarter at an angle, right above where you see the core, and voilà, the core is removed.

Make sure you are using a sharp knife. Apples tend to be juicy, which means they can be slippery. It's important to hold the apple in place firmly while keeping your fingertips tucked under.

TROUBLESHOOTING MISTAKES

Apples will begin to oxidize or turn brown as soon as the flesh is exposed to air. Once you peel an apple, it's best to use it immediately or coat it with lemon juice to slow down the oxidation process.

How to Cut an Onion

Onions confound newer cooks because of their many layers. But there is a method to their madness, and cutting them will soon become a breeze if you follow these best practices.

BEST PRACTICES

When cutting onions, it's best to use a sharp chef's knife. Be sure to hold the onion firmly and curl your fingertips under to prevent injury.

To slice: Begin by slicing ¼ inch from the stem end (not the root end). Halve the onion through the root. Place the cut sides down on the cutting board. Carefully peel back the skin layer from each half. To slice the onion, make crosswise cuts to the desired thickness. If you're only using one half in your recipe, leave the skin on the unused half, tightly wrap it in plastic wrap or in a resealable bag, and place it in the refrigerator for up to 2 weeks.

To dice: Halve the onion through the root. Make lengthwise cuts with the knife tip starting about ⅛ inch from the root end and cutting all the way through the stem end. The number of cuts depends on the size of the onion and the dice you want. Next, hold the onion firmly in place with your fingertips curled under, and slice the onion crosswise, beginning at the stem end and working toward the root end. Start the cut at the root end, because you want to make sure you don't accidentally cut through the root end.

TROUBLESHOOTING MISTAKES

The good thing is, it's hard to mess up when cutting an onion. But you can have a good cry. To minimize eye burning, keep the cut side of the onion on the cutting board so the gasses won't waft up to your eyes. You can also rinse the onion under cold water to remove the enzymes that cause eye discomfort.

How to Mince Garlic

If you find yourself mincing garlic a lot, you may want to invest in a garlic press. Garlic presses produce a consistent mince every time, and many times, you don't even need to peel the cloves. If you prefer an even finer mince, you can grate peeled garlic cloves with a zester.

BEST PRACTICES

To mince garlic, begin by placing the whole garlic bulb on a cutting board with the root side down. Using your palm, press down on the top to loosen the cloves. Separate the number of cloves that you need.

Next, trim off the tip and the root end from each clove you want to mince. Place the flat part of a chef's knife, with the blade facing away from you, on top of a single clove and press down firmly to loosen the skin, then remove the skin.

Cut the cloves into thin slices, then run the knife crosswise across the slices until the garlic is finely chopped. With the tip of the knife on the cutting board, rock the knife up and down in a fan shape to mince the garlic to the desired size.

When using fresh garlic in a recipe, it's best to mince it right before cooking. When garlic flesh is exposed to air, the flavor will change. When you cook with fresh minced garlic, it's best to add it after other aromatics (like onions, peppers, and carrots) have already softened. Garlic, especially minced garlic, will burn quickly, resulting in a bitter taste.

TROUBLESHOOTING MISTAKES

If you accidentally mince more garlic than you need, you can easily store it for later. Simply place it in a small container, cover the minced garlic with olive oil, secure a tight-fitting lid, and refrigerate. It will be good to use for the next 2 to 3 days.

Classic Tossed Salad with Homemade Vinaigrette

Serves 4	**Prep time:** 10 minutes

Skills used: Dicing, mincing, peeling, shredding

2 romaine hearts, chopped
1 medium English cucumber, peeled and diced
2 small Roma tomatoes, diced
½ small red onion, thinly sliced
1 carrot, shredded
¼ cup extra-virgin olive oil
2 tablespoons red wine vinegar
1 teaspoon Dijon mustard
1 garlic clove, very finely minced
1 teaspoon honey
¼ teaspoon table salt
Freshly ground black pepper

Per Serving: Calories: 210; Fat: 15g; Saturated fat: 2g; Cholesterol: 0mg; Carbohydrates: 19g; Fiber: 8g; Protein: 5g; Sodium: 200mg

Everyone should have a go-to salad and homemade dressing in their arsenal. This crisp option is topped with a bright and flavorful vinaigrette. You can easily change up the flavor by swapping in different types of vinegar, such as balsamic. You can even make this salad a hearty meal by adding a cooked protein, such as shrimp, salmon, or slices of Perfect Roast Chicken (page 86).

1. In a large salad bowl, combine the lettuce with the cucumber, tomatoes, onion, and carrot. Use tongs to toss the salad.

2. In a small container with a tight-fitting lid, combine the olive oil, vinegar, mustard, garlic, honey, salt, and a pinch of pepper. Put the lid on the container, and shake vigorously until the dressing is combined.

3. Just before serving, pour the desired amount of dressing over the portion of the salad that you plan to eat immediately, and toss again until everything is coated.

4. To store undressed leftover salad, place the salad in a container, add a single layer of paper towel to absorb excess moisture, and attach a tight-fitting lid. Salad is best when used within 1 to 2 days. Store leftover dressing in a small container with a tight-fitting lid for up to 4 days.

VARIATION TIP: You can add any of your favorite vegetables or toppings, such as sliced olives, drained and rinsed chickpeas, or croutons.

Mashed Potatoes in a Snap

| Serves 6 | **Prep time:** 10 minutes | **Cook time:** 20 minutes |

Skills used: Chopping, boiling, measuring, knife skills, mashing

3 pounds russet potatoes, peeled and chopped into 1-inch pieces

2 teaspoons table salt, divided

¼ cup (½ stick) unsalted butter

¼ cup sour cream

⅔ cup half-and-half

⅛ teaspoon freshly ground black pepper

Per Serving: Calories: 301; Fat: 13g; Saturated fat: 8g; Cholesterol: 35mg; Carbohydrates: 42g; Fiber: 3g; Protein: 6g; Sodium: 803mg

Who doesn't want to master this crowd-pleaser? No more flaky boxed mashed potatoes for you. In just half an hour, you can have your own creamy, buttery, delectable version. Just a tip, make sure you check the potatoes for doneness and remove them as soon as they are fork-tender, because overcooking them makes them mealy, an unpleasant texture.

1. In a large pot, cover the chopped potatoes with cold water. Add 1 teaspoon salt. Cover the pot, and bring it to a boil over high heat. Once boiling, reduce the heat to medium-high, and continue to boil potatoes for about 15 minutes or until cooked through. You can tell if they're done by sticking a fork into one of the pieces. If it comes out easily, the potatoes are done. Drain the potatoes, and put them in a large bowl.

2. Add the butter, sour cream, and remaining 1 teaspoon salt. Use a potato masher or electric beaters to mash the potatoes until no lumps remain. Slowly stir in the half-and-half until the mashed potatoes reach the desired consistency. Stir in the pepper, taste, and add more salt if needed.

3. To store leftovers, allow the mashed potatoes to cool completely, place them in a container with a tight-fitting lid, and refrigerate for up to 4 days.

GENERAL TIP: It might seem easier to use a food processor or blender to mash the potatoes, but using these methods will release too much starch and make the mashed potatoes sticky and gluey.

Robust Roasted Root Vegetables

| Serves 4 | **Prep time:** 20 minutes | **Cook time:** 35 minutes |

Skills used: Chopping, mincing, roasting, knife skills

Nonstick cooking spray
1 large sweet potato, peeled and chopped into 1½-inch pieces
3 to 4 medium red potatoes, chopped into 1½-inch pieces
2 medium beets peeled and chopped into 1½-inch pieces
2 large carrots, peeled and chopped into 1½-inch pieces
1 medium parsnip, peeled and chopped into 1½-inch pieces
½ red onion, chopped into 1½-inch pieces
4 garlic cloves, minced
2 tablespoons minced fresh thyme leaves
2 tablespoons minced fresh rosemary
¼ cup extra-virgin olive oil
1 teaspoon table salt
¼ teaspoon freshly ground black pepper

Per Serving: Calories: 329; Fat: 14g; Saturated fat: 2g; Cholesterol: 0mg; Carbohydrates: 48g; Fiber: 8g; Protein: 5g; Sodium: 690mg

Root vegetables are those that grow beneath the soil. They are just packed with nutrients including fiber; antioxidants; potassium; vitamins A, B, and C; and the list goes on. Simply roasting them with some herbs in a hot oven brings out their natural sweetness and earthy tones, making them a perfect side dish for any main course; serve them instead of fries with the Grilled Bacon Cheeseburger (page 98).

1. Place the oven rack on the lowest position in the oven. Preheat the oven to 400°F. Prepare a rimmed baking sheet by spraying it with cooking spray.

2. In a large bowl, combine the sweet and red potatoes, beets, carrots, parsnip, and onion. Add the garlic, thyme, and rosemary, as well as the olive oil. Stir until fully combined.

3. Spread the vegetables onto the rimmed baking sheet, making sure that they are in a single layer. Sprinkle the salt and pepper on them.

4. Roast the vegetables for 15 minutes. Stir well, and return them to the oven for 20 additional minutes. The vegetables are done when you can stick a fork into the center of each type, and the fork goes through without resistance.

5. To store leftovers, allow them to cool completely, place them in a container with a tight-fitting lid, and refrigerate for up to 4 days.

FLAVOR BOOST TIP: Amp up the flavor of this side dish by tossing the veggies with a splash of balsamic vinegar during the last few minutes of roasting.

Rainbow Stir-Fry

| Serves 4 | **Prep time:** 10 minutes | **Cook time:** 10 minutes |

Skills used: Mincing, sautéing, slicing, knife skills, measuring

½ cup chicken broth
¼ cup soy sauce
3 garlic cloves, minced
3 tablespoons packed light brown sugar
1 tablespoon cornstarch
1 teaspoon sesame oil
1 tablespoon extra-virgin olive oil
2 bell peppers (varied colors), seeded and sliced
2 cups broccoli florets (from 1 head broccoli)
1 cup sugar snap peas, ends and strings removed
1 cup sliced carrots
1 cup sliced white button mushrooms
½ cup canned water chestnuts, drained

Per Serving: Calories: 189; Fat: 6g; Saturated fat: 1g; Cholesterol: 0mg; Carbohydrates: 31g; Fiber: 6g; Protein: 6g; Sodium: 920mg

This crispy, flavorful stir-fry is just right for a healthy, wholesome dinner, and it's ready in less time than take-out or delivery. Be sure not to over-sauté the veggies because they will lose their crispness. Make it heartier, but no less healthy, by adding a lean protein such as shrimp (I'm partial to the Sticky Honey Garlic Shrimp on page 66) or serving it over cooked brown rice (see How to Cook Rice, page 31).

1. In a small bowl, whisk together the chicken broth, soy sauce, garlic, brown sugar, cornstarch, and sesame oil. Set aside.

2. Heat a large skillet over medium-high heat, and pour in the olive oil. Add the bell peppers, broccoli, sugar snap peas, carrots, and mushrooms. Sauté for 3 minutes, or until crisp-tender. The vegetables will start to soften slightly but will still have a crisp snap to them. Add the water chestnuts, and pour the sauce mixture over the vegetables. Sauté for 3 to 5 minutes or until the sauce has thickened.

3. To store leftovers, allow the stir-fry to cool completely, place it in a container with a tight-fitting lid, and refrigerate for up to 4 days.

INGREDIENT TIP: You can easily swap frozen veggies for fresh in this recipe. Thaw 2 (12-ounce) bags of frozen stir-fry vegetables, drain off any excess water and pat the veggies dry with paper towels. Sauté the veggies for 2 to 3 minutes until heated through and crisp-tender.

Easy as Apple Crisp

| Serves 4 | **Prep time:** 20 minutes | **Cook time:** 45 minutes |

Skills used: Peeling, coring, chopping, baking

5 cups peeled, cored, sliced Honeycrisp apples (about 7 medium apples) (see Variation Tip)
½ cup granulated sugar
½ cup plus ½ tablespoon all-purpose flour, divided
½ teaspoon ground cinnamon
2 tablespoons water
½ cup quick oats
½ cup packed light brown sugar
⅛ teaspoon baking powder
⅛ teaspoon baking soda
¼ cup unsalted butter, melted

Per Serving: Calories: 488; Fat: 13g; Saturated fat: 8g; Cholesterol: 31mg; Carbohydrates: 92g; Fiber: 4g; Protein: 5g; Sodium: 63mg

We can't forget that fruits and veggies have a super-fun side. This classic apple crisp will be sure to impress any guests and comfort you on a chilly evening. It's easy to make and can be served warm or cold. Make it even more decadent by adding a scoop of vanilla ice cream.

1. Preheat the oven to 350°F.
2. In an 8-inch square baking dish, spread out the apple slices.
3. In a medium bowl, combine the sugar, ½ tablespoon flour, and the cinnamon, and stir to combine. Sprinkle the sugar mixture evenly over the apples. Pour the water into the baking dish.
4. In a medium bowl, combine ½ cup of flour and the quick oats, brown sugar, baking powder, and baking soda. Stir until combined. Pour the melted butter over the oat mixture, and stir until the mixture becomes crumbly. Spread the crumb mixture out evenly over the apples.
5. Bake for 45 minutes. When finished, the apples should be tender, and the juices will be bubbling around the edges.
6. To store leftovers, allow the crisp to cool completely, and cover the baking dish tightly with plastic wrap. Refrigerate for up to 3 days.

VARIATION TIP: For a fun twist, replace the apples with an equal amount of peeled, cored, and sliced pears. Or experiment with different types of apples.

Fruits and Vegetables

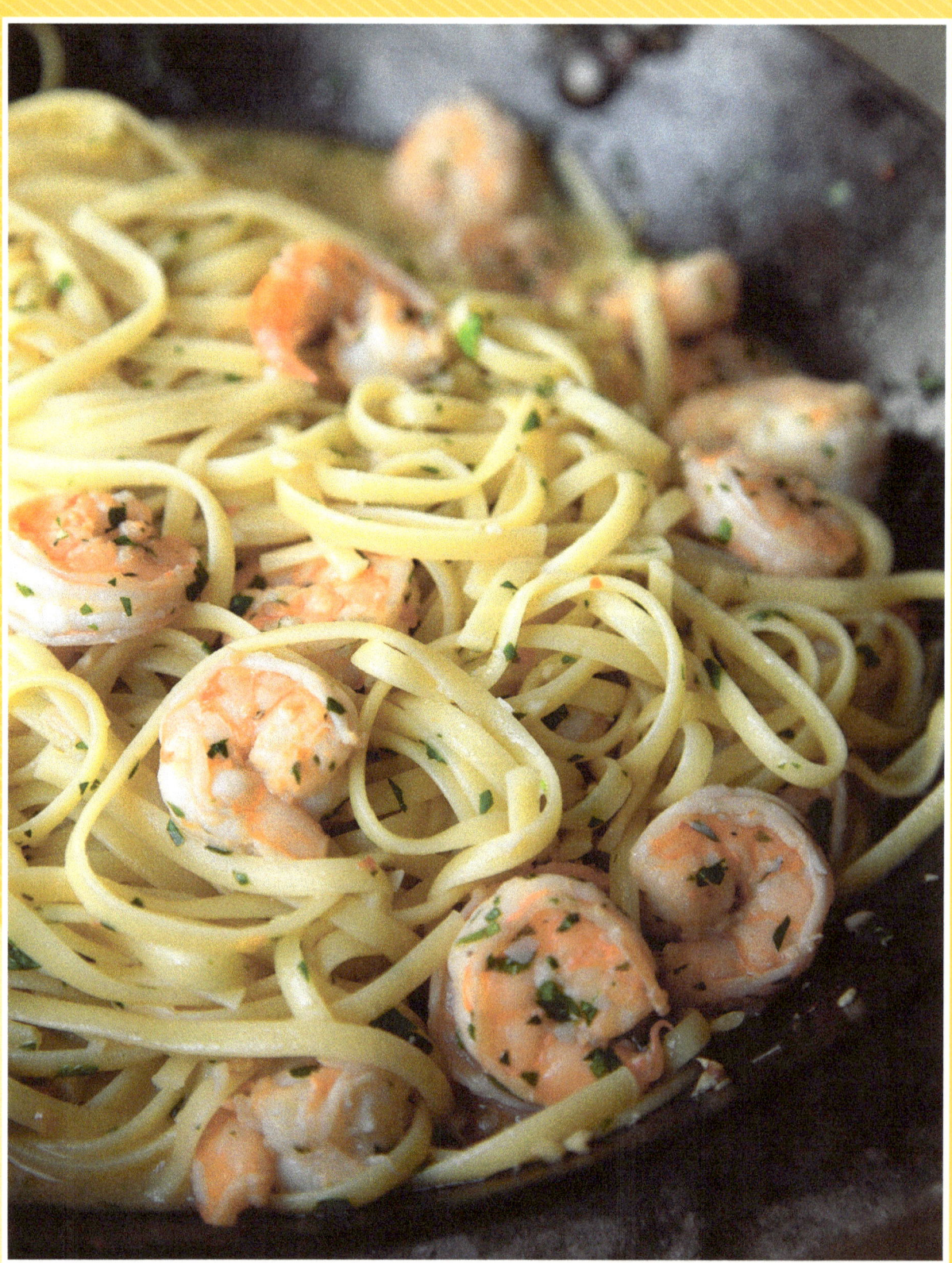

Simple Scrumptious Shrimp Scampi, page 64.

CHAPTER 5

Seafood

There is a vast array of seafood to suit all different tastes and diets, and it can be prepared in so many ways. Seafood can seem intimidating, but you'll find that it's just as easy as cooking other proteins. In this chapter, you'll learn about types of seafood, purchasing seafood, essential techniques, and some basic preparations.

Simple Scrumptious Shrimp Scampi 64

Sticky Honey Garlic Shrimp 66

Soy-Ginger Scallops 67

Lemon Butter Fish Packets 68

Coconut Curry Salmon 70

Plenty of Fish

When it comes to fish and seafood, there is so much available, even if you're landlocked. Fish and seafood are great for beginners, because they don't require fancy cooking techniques. You can quickly prepare delicious and healthy meals using simple techniques, such as searing, grilling, steaming, and baking.

You'll find a good variety of fresh seafood and fish in most grocery stores. You can also find quality frozen options, which are just as good as fresh because most are frozen right after harvest. Some stores even employ fishmongers, professionals trained to handle, bone, fillet, and sell fish and seafood.

Fish and seafood can spoil quickly, so give it a sniff before preparing it. When shopping for seafood and fish, it should have a mild smell that's briny and fresh. Fresh fish and seafood will not have a strong fishy odor.

FISH

There are many types of fish available, both saltwater and freshwater varieties. Fish are often grouped by texture—delicate, medium, and firm. Delicate fish include choices like flounder, anchovies, and mackerel. The medium-textured variety includes cod, tilapia, sea bass, and salmon. Catfish, halibut, swordfish, and tuna are firmer-textured options.

Fish can be purchased whole or already filleted. For a beginner cook, filleted fish is an easier option because the head is off, and the flesh has been separated from the bone. Fillets can come with or without skin.

When selecting fish, it's important to notice the smell and to choose bright-colored fish. If you're purchasing fillets, look for vibrant-colored flesh or skin. Avoid fish that is dull or discolored. Some fish may have a clear liquid on the flesh. If the liquid is milky colored, it's not fresh. Fresh fish will also spring back when you press on the flesh. If you press on the meat and your finger leaves an indent that doesn't bounce back, it's not fresh. If you're purchasing whole fish, look at the eyes. They should be clear with a slight bulge.

The price of fish can vary greatly, depending on the type and your region. As with most fresh foods, fish sourced locally will be more affordable than fish brought in from other regions. Also, white-fleshed fish, such as cod, tilapia, bass, and grouper, is typically more affordable. Frozen fish is also a great option for beginner cooks (see Smoked, Canned, and Frozen Seafood, page 59).

You can cook fish in several ways, including sautéing, panfrying, grilling, and broiling. When cooking fish, you can easily tell when it's done using a meat thermometer. The temperature should be 145°F. The fish will have an opaque color and will easily flake apart with a fork. It's important to note that fish cooks fast, so always start checking the temperature at the minimum cooking time for the recipe.

SHELLFISH

The most common shellfish and crustaceans include scallops, shrimp, crabs, lobster, clams, oysters, and mussels. When buying shellfish and crustaceans, it's important to smell them. They should smell briny and like the sea, not "fishy." When purchasing fresh seafood from the fish counter, you can ask to smell it and inspect it before it's wrapped up for purchase. Fresh shellfish and crustaceans do not have a long shelf life. It's best to use them within one day of purchase.

You can also purchase a lot of shellfish frozen. This is a great option if you don't live in a region with easy access to fresh seafood. These are frozen at harvest to preserve the freshness and moisture. One of the benefits of the frozen variety is you can thaw just the amount you need and leave the rest frozen, eliminating waste.

Purchasing shellfish and crustaceans can be pricey, depending on the type. Like everything else, shellfish and crustaceans are most affordable when purchased in season and sourced locally. It's also smart to look for sales and nab them when they're cheaper (and freeze them, if you can). Mussels generally are the most affordable.

Shellfish and crustaceans are versatile proteins that can be cooked in a number of ways. Common preparations include steaming, broiling, poaching, and grilling. Like fish, shellfish and crustaceans should be cooked to an internal temperature of 145°F. Some seafood, such as lobster, is easier to check with a thermometer. For other varieties, you need to rely on visual cues. When shellfish like shrimp and crabs are fully cooked, they will turn opaque, and the color will turn from gray to pink. Crustaceans, such as clams and mussels, should be fully open.

SMOKED, CANNED, AND FROZEN SEAFOOD

One of the great things about seafood is it can easily be preserved to increase its shelf life. There are three main types: smoked, canned, and frozen.

Smoked seafood is salted, then cured with smoke. The process draws out the moisture and leaves a denser, more flavorful meat. The most common types of smoked seafood are salmon, trout, whitefish, and mackerel. Smoked fish should have a bright color. If you notice a slimy film or sour odor, these are signs that the fish is bad. Smoked fish is a great addition to salads, pasta, dips, or simply atop a bagel. It can last up to 3 weeks in the refrigerator.

Canning is another economical way to preserve seafood. Tuna is the most common type of canned seafood, but you can also find canned crab, shrimp, clams, sardines, salmon, anchovies, and herring, to name a few. Canned seafood has a longer shelf life than other varieties. Always check the sell-by or best-by date on the can before using canned seafood. Both smoked and canned seafood can be used straight from the package; they don't need to be cooked.

Freezing is another way to preserve the shelf life of seafood. This is a cost-effective alternative to fresh seafood, and the quality is just as good because it's often frozen right on the boat as soon as it's caught. This ensures that the seafood is preserved at the peak of freshness. In fact, much of the "fresh" seafood you see in a grocery store was previously frozen. When buying frozen seafood, look for packages that do not have ice crystals or frost. Also, avoid frozen seafood that isn't frozen solid.

Prepping Seafood

When working with seafood, make sure it's always kept cold. When traveling home from the market, keep seafood on ice. Once you get it home, it's best to use it within one day.

The first step in working with seafood is proper cleaning. Fish and seafood contain things like bones, scales, and sand, all of which make for a disappointing and even dangerous (bones) dining experience. Always use cold water when rinsing seafood. Using warm water can cause bacteria to form. Thoroughly scrub the shells of crustaceans, such as clams and mussels, to remove any grit. Mussels also have thin threads attached to the shell called a "beard." Use a knife to remove the beard from the shell carefully. This is also a great time to inspect crustaceans for broken shells; throw out any that have broken shells.

Once the seafood is cleaned, use paper towels to blot off excess moisture. This is especially important if you're searing or broiling. Surface moisture will cause the seafood to steam when cooked and prevent it from browning. When drying the seafood, inspect and remove any pin bones (thin bones found in fish) and pieces of shell or grit.

Whether using salt and pepper or a blend of herbs and spices, it's important to season the seafood liberally early on. Also, because it's so lean, seafood tends to stick to the pan when it is being cooked. Be sure to use butter, oil, or nonstick cooking spray to ensure the seafood releases from the pan or cooking surface.

How to Thaw Frozen Seafood

Frozen fish and shellfish are an affordable and accessible alternative to fresh seafood. Because fish and seafood are delicate proteins that tend to spoil quickly, it's important you thaw them properly.

BEST PRACTICES

To thaw frozen seafood, soak it in cold water. If the seafood is in a plastic package, place the package in a container of cold water, making sure it's completely submerged. If it's wrapped in butcher paper, transfer it to a zip-top bag and submerge it in cold water. If needed, place a dinner plate on top of the package to ensure that it's fully submerged. Change the water every 30 minutes until the seafood is thawed. Once it's defrosted, remove the seafood from the package, and cook it immediately. Frozen shellfish, such as shrimp and scallops, often come in large packages. If you only need to use a portion of the package, separate the frozen shellfish into individual portions and place each in a zip-top bag. Seal the bag(s), making sure you remove any excess air, and label with the contents, amount, and date. Return the bags you're not thawing immediately to the freezer. It's important that the seafood does not thaw while you are repackaging, so you need to work quickly.

TROUBLESHOOTING MISTAKES

If the seafood thaws inadvertently, check for freshness before preparing it. If it's still cold and the color and smell are good, you can cook the seafood, but do it immediately.

How to Peel and Devein Shrimp

Buying shrimp with the shell on is more affordable than the peeled and deveined variety. This outer shell needs to be removed before eating, and the dark vein, the shrimp's gritty digestive tract that runs down the back of the shrimp, should be removed, as well. Peeling and deveining shrimp can seem intimidating for a beginner cook, but it's really quite easy.

BEST PRACTICES

The easiest way to peel and devein is to use kitchen shears. Shallowly cut along the top of the shell, stopping when you get to the tail. Peel back the shell and discard. If you want to remove the tail, find where it meets the body, gently pinch, and pull it away. If you don't have kitchen shears, you can use your fingers.

Once the shell is removed, use a paring knife to make a shallow cut along the back of the shrimp to expose the vein. Use the tip of the knife to gently pull up on the vein and remove it. Not all shrimp have veins.

TROUBLESHOOTING MISTAKES

Sometimes, when deveining shrimp, the vein can break as you remove it. When this happens, use the tip of a paring knife to remove the remaining sections. Also, it is not necessary to remove the veins. It is personal preference, but they can be unsightly, gritty, and unpleasant to eat.

How to Cook Fish in a Foil Packet

Cooking fish in a foil packet is an easy way to steam fish to tender perfection. This cooking method is just like it sounds. You wrap fish, seasonings, and other ingredients in a piece of aluminum foil and bake it. The fish steams and is infused with the flavors in the packet. No mess, no fish smell in your kitchen, and everyone can make their own custom packet.

BEST PRACTICES

Start by choosing your favorite veggies; tender vegetables, such as green beans, bell peppers, zucchini, asparagus, onions, and thin carrot slices, work best. Layer one cup of vegetables on a piece of aluminum foil (sprayed with nonstick cooking spray) and top with one portion of fish (about 3 ounces), such as tilapia, halibut, or cod. Sprinkle ½ to 1½ teaspoons of your favorite seasoning blend over the top. I like to make a mixture of ½ teaspoon salt, ½ teaspoon Italian seasoning blend, ¼ teaspoon garlic powder, and ⅛ teaspoon pepper. You can also add fresh aromatics, such as lemon slices, garlic cloves, or fresh herbs. Drizzle 2 tablespoons of melted butter over the top, and wrap the foil up tightly, ensuring no gaps for the liquid to drip out. Bake the packet at 350°F for 15 to 20 minutes.

I prefer to place the foil packets on a rimmed baking sheet before adding the ingredients. The rimmed baking sheet is a great way to contain leaks and keep your oven clean.

TROUBLESHOOTING MISTAKES

If you open the packet and the fish isn't cooked through, quickly close the packet back up and return it to the oven until the fish reaches an internal temperature of 145°F. Remember, though, every time you open the packet, you release the steam needed to cook the fish.

Simple Scrumptious Shrimp Scampi

| Serves 6 | **Prep time:** 10 minutes | **Cook time:** 15 minutes |

Skills used: Knife skills, measuring, sautéing, peeling and deveining shrimp, mincing

1 pound linguine
¼ cup (½ stick) unsalted butter, divided
¼ cup extra-virgin olive oil, divided
4 garlic cloves, minced
1 shallot, minced
⅛ teaspoon red pepper flakes
1 pound large or extra-large shrimp, peeled and deveined (See General Tip)
¾ teaspoon table salt
⅛ teaspoon freshly ground black pepper
½ cup dry white wine (see Simple Rice Pilaf, Tips, page 39)
Juice of 1 lemon
⅓ cup chopped fresh parsley

Per Serving: Calories: 515; Fat: 18g; Saturated fat: 6g; Cholesterol: 142mg; Carbohydrates: 59g; Fiber: 3g; Protein: 25g; Sodium: 450mg

Shrimp scampi is one of my favorite dishes to make. This buttery, garlicky, pasta-y recipe sounds impressive to guests but is surprisingly easy to make for cooks at all levels. Plus, it only takes about 25 minutes from start to finish. Amp up the citrus flavor by quartering the juiced lemon and placing the quarters into the skillet when you add the shrimp.

1. Bring a large pot of salted water to a boil. When the water has come to a full boil, add the linguine, and cook according to the package directions (see How to Cook Pasta, page 30).

2. While the linguine is cooking, in a large skillet, melt 2 tablespoons of the butter and warm 2 tablespoons of the olive oil over medium-high heat. Add the garlic, shallot, and red pepper flakes, and sauté for 3 minutes or until the shallot is translucent.

3. While the shallot cooks, season the shrimp with salt and pepper. Add the seasoned shrimp to the pan, and cook until they turn pink, about 3 minutes.

4. Remove the shrimp from the skillet with tongs or a slotted spoon and set them aside on a plate.

5. Add the wine and lemon juice to the skillet, and bring it to a light boil. Add the remaining 2 tablespoons of butter and olive oil, and whisk until the butter is melted. Add the shrimp back to the skillet, and toss to coat. Turn off the heat.

6. Drain the linguine, and add it to the skillet. Stir in the parsley, and toss until everything is completely coated. Taste for seasoning, and add additional salt and pepper if needed.

7. To store leftovers, allow the dish to cool completely, place it in a container with a tight-fitting lid, and refrigerate for up to 2 days.

GENERAL TIP: Don't throw those shrimp shells away. You can use them to make a quick and delicious stock that works as a base for other dishes, such as Creamy Risotto (page 36). In a large saucepan, melt 1 tablespoon butter over medium-high heat. When the butter has melted, add the shells from 1 pound of shrimp, along with a quartered onion, chopped carrot, chopped celery stalk, and 2 smashed garlic cloves. Cook for 10 minutes, or until the shrimp shells are pink and the vegetables soften. Add 2 cups of water, 1 bay leaf, and 1 teaspoon black peppercorns. Bring to a boil, reduce the heat, and simmer for 10 minutes. Strain the broth into a container and discard all the solids. You can store it in the refrigerator for up to 4 days or freeze for up to 3 months.

Sticky Honey Garlic Shrimp

Serves 4	**Prep time:** 5 minutes, plus 30 minutes to marinate	**Cook time:** 10 minutes

Skills used: Measuring, peeling and deveining shrimp, mincing

½ cup honey
¼ cup soy sauce
3 garlic cloves, minced
1 tablespoon peeled and grated fresh ginger, from 1-inch piece
Juice from 1 lemon
1 pound large or extra-large shrimp, peeled and deveined (see Simple Scrumptious Shrimp Scampi, General Tip, page 65)
2 tablespoons unsalted butter

Per Serving: Calories: 221; Fat: 6g; Saturated fat: 4g; Cholesterol: 198mg; Carbohydrates: 19g; Fiber: 0g; Protein: 24g; Sodium: 576mg

This shrimp dish is incredibly flavorful and versatile, and is a truly healthy choice, especially served over cooked brown rice, with a side of steamed broccoli or green beans, or on top of a salad. It also makes a great appetizer. If you have any leftovers, reheat them in a small skillet for 1 to 2 minutes and then add them as protein to the Veggie Ramen Bowl (page 42).

1. In a small bowl, whisk the honey, soy sauce, garlic, ginger, and lemon juice until combined.

2. In a large bowl, place the shrimp. Pour half the sauce over the shrimp, and let it marinate in the refrigerator for 30 minutes. Set the remaining half of the sauce aside.

3. In a medium skillet, melt the butter over medium-high heat. When the butter has melted, add the marinated shrimp, discarding the marinade it was soaking in.

4. Cook for about 2 minutes, then flip the shrimp, and cook for an additional 2 minutes or until the shrimp turn pink. Pour the reserved marinade from step 2 over the shrimp, and cook for 1 to 2 minutes until the sauce thickens slightly.

5. To store leftovers, allow the dish to cool completely, place it in a container with a tight-fitting lid, and refrigerate for up to 2 days.

TROUBLESHOOTING TIP: Shrimp only need a few minutes to cook through. Shrimp are cooked when they are uniformly pink and opaque, with no gray spots.

Soy-Ginger Scallops

| Serves 4 | **Prep time:** 10 minutes | **Cook time:** 20 minutes |

Skills used: Mincing, measuring, baking

1½ pounds large fresh, or frozen and thawed, scallops
¼ cup extra-virgin olive oil
¼ cup soy sauce
¼ cup peeled and grated fresh ginger, from 4-inch piece
4 garlic cloves, minced
1 teaspoon red pepper flakes

Per Serving: Calories: 254; Fat: 14g; Saturated fat: 2g; Cholesterol: 41mg; Carbohydrates: 8g; Fiber: 0g; Protein: 22g; Sodium: 1,544mg

Scallops have a delicate texture and a rich taste with a slight sweetness that make them delicious. You can show off for guests with this seemingly impressive but really quick and easy, dish. The key is to make sure the scallops don't overcook. Baking them is a gentler way of cooking so they don't turn rubbery. If you're using frozen scallops, make sure they are fully thawed before cooking. You can serve them with a side of rice and Robust Roasted Root Vegetables (page 53) or atop the Classic Tossed Salad with Homemade Vinaigrette (page 51) or add them as protein to the Rainbow Stir-Fry (page 54).

1. Preheat the oven to 450°F.
2. Rinse the scallops, pat them dry, and arrange them in a single layer in a 9-inch square baking dish.
3. In a small bowl, combine the olive oil, soy sauce, ginger, garlic, and red pepper flakes. Pour the sauce over the scallops.
4. Bake for 15 to 20 minutes or until the internal temperature reaches 120°F on a meat thermometer. The scallops will be opaque when they are cooked through.
5. To store leftovers, allow them to cool completely, place them in a container with a tight-fitting lid, and refrigerate for up to 2 days.

GENERAL TIP: If you'd like to get a head start on this recipe, make the sauce up to 8 hours before you bake the scallops.

Lemon Butter Fish Packets

| Serves 4 | **Prep time:** 15 minutes | **Cook time:** 20 minutes |

Skills used: Knife skills, measuring, cooking in foil packets, mincing, slicing

- 1 medium yellow onion, thinly sliced
- ½ pound fresh green beans, trimmed (see Ingredient Tip)
- 1 teaspoon table salt, divided
- ½ teaspoon freshly ground black pepper, divided
- 1 tablespoon extra-virgin olive oil
- 4 (4-ounce) whitefish fillets, such as tilapia or cod
- 2 tablespoons unsalted butter, melted
- 3 garlic cloves, minced
- ¼ teaspoon red pepper flakes
- 1 lemon, thinly sliced into 8 pieces

Per Serving: Calories: 222; Fat: 11g; Saturated fat: 5g; Cholesterol: 72mg; Carbohydrates: 7g; Fiber: 2g; Protein: 24g; Sodium: 646mg

Easy and delicious, this whole meal can be prepped and cooked in close to 30 minutes. I recommend using whitefish for this recipe because it is generally mild and cooks quickly. Cod is a sweeter option, and full of flavor, and tilapia is a more sustainable choice, very mild, with just a slight sweetness. Whatever you choose, give it a boost with Simple Rice Pilaf (page 38).

1. Preheat the oven to 400°F.
2. Tear aluminum foil into four 15-inch pieces. Evenly divide the onion slices between the four pieces, placing them in the center of each foil sheet.
3. In a medium bowl, mix the green beans with ½ teaspoon salt and ⅛ teaspoon pepper. Drizzle with the olive oil, and toss to combine. Divide the green beans among the foil packets on top of the onions.
4. Place a fish fillet on top of the green beans on each foil sheet.
5. In a small bowl, combine the melted butter, garlic, remaining ½ teaspoon salt, ⅜ teaspoon pepper, and the red pepper flakes. Stir to combine, and evenly divide it over the fish fillets. Place two lemon slices on top of each fish fillet.

6. Fold the foil over the fish, and tightly wrap it. Fold each end up to prevent any liquid from escaping. Place the packets on rimmed baking sheets (two packets per sheet). After about 18 minutes, insert a meat thermometer through the top of the foil packet into the fish. Continue testing at 1-minute increments until the internal temperature of the fish reaches 145°F on a meat thermometer.

7. To store leftovers, allow the packets to cool completely, place them in a container with a tight-fitting lid, and refrigerate for up to 2 days.

FLAVOR BOOST TIP: You can easily kick up the flavor of these fish packets by adding your favorite herbs. Try adding ⅛ teaspoon dried dill or thyme per packet.

INGREDIENT TIP: This recipe uses fresh green beans, but you can easily substitute frozen green beans. Thaw them and drain off any excess water before seasoning and adding them to the foil packets.

Coconut Curry Salmon

| Serves 4 | **Prep time:** 5 minutes | **Cook time:** 30 minutes |

Skills used: Slicing, mincing, measuring, cooking rice

- 4 (4-ounce) skin-on salmon fillets
- 1 teaspoon table salt
- ½ teaspoon freshly ground black pepper
- 1 tablespoon canola oil
- 1 shallot, thinly sliced
- 1 tablespoon red curry paste (see Ingredient Tip)
- 2 garlic cloves, minced
- 2 teaspoons peeled and grated fresh ginger, from ½-inch piece
- 1 (14-ounce) can coconut milk
- 1 tablespoon sriracha
- 1 tablespoon fish sauce
- 3 cups cooked rice, for serving (see How to Cook Rice, page 31)
- 4 lime wedges, for serving
- Fresh cilantro, chopped, for serving

Per Serving: Calories: 584; Fat: 31g; Saturated fat: 20g; Cholesterol: 51mg; Carbohydrates: 45g; Fiber: 1g; Protein: 30g; Sodium: 1,001mg

Coconut curry salmon is a quick, simple, healthy recipe that features delicious flavors from the coconut milk, red curry paste, and a touch of sriracha for heat. This recipe uses salmon fillets with the skin on. When cooking salmon with skin, it's important to keep the skin as crispy as possible. This is why you should place the salmon, skin-side up, into the sauce. If you prefer the texture of skinless salmon, you can buy skinless fillets or remove the skin yourself.

1. Season the salmon with the salt and pepper. In a large skillet, heat the oil over medium-high heat. When the oil is hot, add the salmon, skin-side down, and cook for 5 minutes. Flip the salmon, and cook for an additional 5 minutes. Transfer it to a plate, and set aside. The salmon is not fully cooked at this point.

2. Return the skillet to the heat, and add the shallot. Cook it for 3 minutes, until soft and translucent. Add the red curry paste, garlic, and ginger to the skillet, and cook for 1 minute, until fragrant.

3. Reduce the heat to medium, and slowly whisk in the coconut milk. Stir in the sriracha and fish sauce, and bring the mixture to a simmer.

4. Add the salmon back to the skillet, skin-side up, and simmer for 15 minutes, stirring occasionally, until the internal temperature of the salmon is 145°F on a meat thermometer.

5. Serve the salmon on top of cooked rice, spoon the sauce on top, and garnish with lime wedges and cilantro.

6. To store leftovers, allow the dish to cool completely, place it in a container with a tight-fitting lid, and refrigerate for up to 2 days.

INGREDIENT TIP: Red curry paste is a traditional Thai ingredient made from red chili peppers, garlic, turmeric, lemongrass, ginger, and salt. It adds a deep, slightly spicy flavor to recipes. You can find red curry paste in the international aisles at most grocery stores.

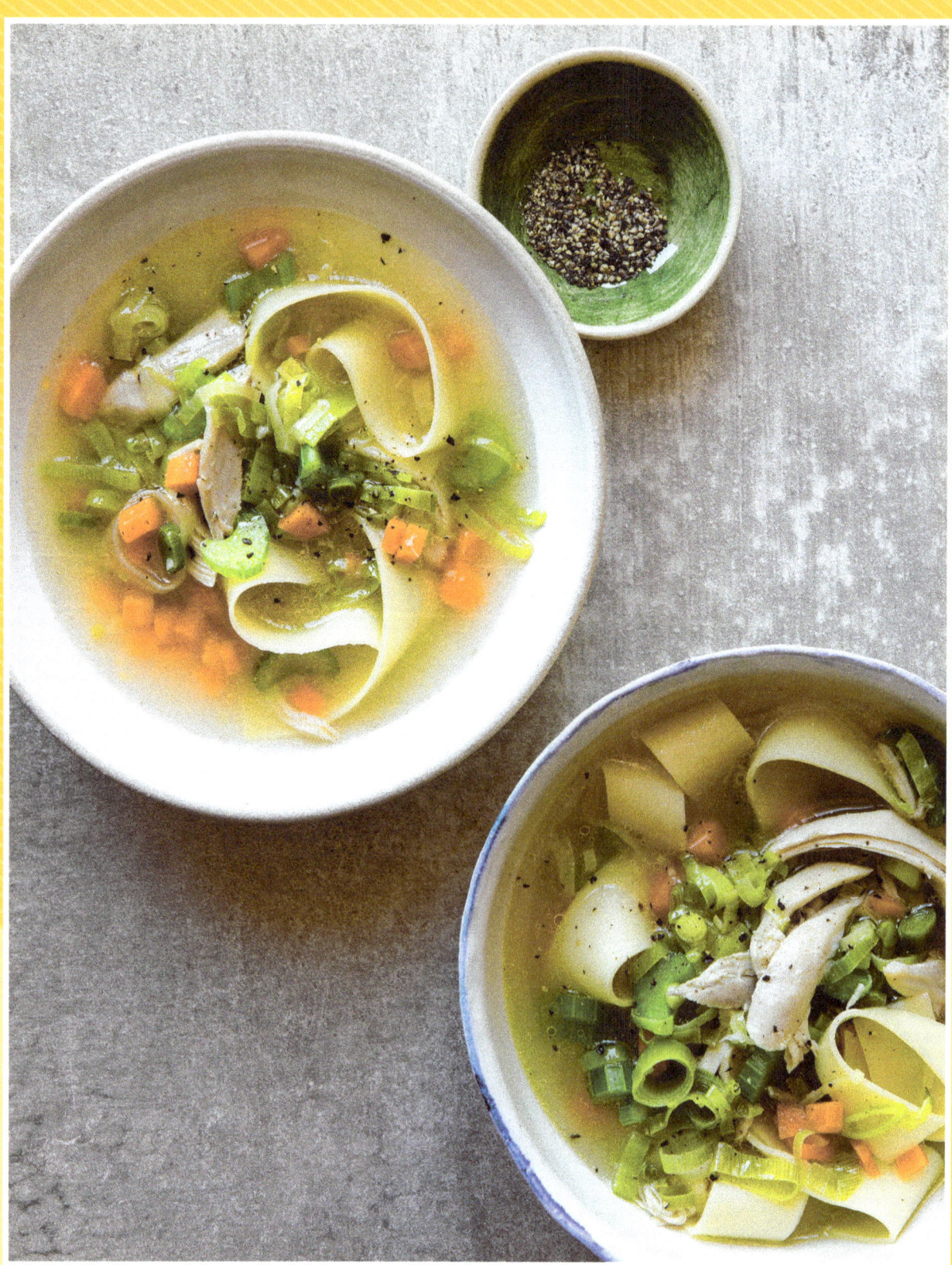

Soothing Chicken Noodle Soup, page 82.

CHAPTER 6

Eggs and Poultry

Poultry and eggs are a staple in most American kitchens, and for a good reason: They're accessible, affordable, easy to prepare, and extremely versatile. This chapter breaks down the most common types of poultry and eggs. You'll learn how and where to buy them, how to store and prepare them, and, most important, how to cook and serve them.

Chicken Cutlets with Lemony Pan Sauce 80

Soothing Chicken Noodle Soup 82

Sheet-Pan Chicken Shawarma 84

Perfect Roast Chicken 86

Denver Omelet 88

Plethora of Poultry

When it comes to poultry, you probably think of chicken and turkey. Duck, geese, guinea fowl, quail, and pigeons also fall under the poultry umbrella, though. Each of these has great flavor, but for the purposes of this book, "poultry" refers to chicken (and their eggs) and turkey.

Poultry can provide high-quality protein with low fat levels. Grocery stores have a wide range of cuts and options, from whole birds to ground meat. You can even buy fresh poultry from local farmers. These versatile proteins have a mild flavor, so they take on the flavors of the dish. Poultry can be grilled, baked, roasted, fried, seared, and poached. The possibilities are endless.

CHICKEN

Grocery stores contain a wide range of chicken options. Chicken is sold whole or broken into parts, including legs, wings, thighs, and breasts. You can find cuts with or without skin and bones. You can even find ground chicken, great for meatballs, burgers, and more. Some chicken parts, such as the legs and thighs, have darker meat, which is more flavorful but higher in fat content. The breasts are white meat, which has a milder flavor and lower fat.

The most affordable cut is chicken leg quarters. This cut consists of the leg and thigh and is sold with the bone in and skin on. Whole chickens are also very affordable when you consider the price per pound. The most expensive cut of chicken is the boneless, skinless chicken breast.

When buying chicken (and turkey), always look at the "best by" date on the package, and select a package that falls within the period of time you'll be cooking it. Also, look at the color of the chicken. It should have a pinkish flesh-colored tint. If the color is dull or grayish, it's probably not fresh. If you're buying chicken with skin, make sure the skin covers the entire piece of meat. When you bring chicken home, store it on the bottom shelf of the refrigerator, so the juices do not come in contact with other foods. It's also important to make sure chicken is fully cooked before serving to avoid any risk of salmonella. Chicken and turkey is cooked through when it reaches an internal temperature of 165°F at their thickest part.

Buy organic? Organic chicken does not contain antibiotics or hormones. The chickens also have the opportunity to roam free, whereas conventional chickens are caged. Studies have shown that organic chickens contain higher omega-3 fatty acids and offer a lower risk for food poisoning.

TURKEY

Turkey is very similar to chicken in taste and texture and only slightly more expensive per pound. Most people only consider turkey during the holiday season; however, it's an economical option whenever you need to feed a crowd. You can usually find turkey in the grocery store throughout the year, not just during the holidays. You're probably familiar with the whole turkey, but you can also get legs, thighs, breasts, and ground turkey. Like chicken, the turkey breasts tend to be more expensive, whereas thighs and legs tend to be more affordable.

Like chicken, when buying turkey, also consider the color. The skin should be a creamy, off-white color, and the meat can range from a purple-ish blue to pink. When turkey is past its prime, the meat will get darker and feel sticky or slimy. Most of the time, we think of roasting a whole turkey, but this meat does well with all types of cooking methods.

EGGS

Eggs are an easy-to-make, protein-rich food. They are used in numerous recipes or eaten on their own. Eggs can be prepared in a number of ways, from soft and hard boiled to poached, sunny-side up, over easy, scrambled, or flip yourself an omelet. The most common eggs are chicken eggs, but you can also cook with quail, duck, and other poultry eggs.

Eggs range in size from jumbo to small. Larger eggs contain more liquid. This is negligible if using one egg, but when a recipe calls for several eggs, the amount of liquid can make a difference. I use large eggs in the recipes.

Different breeds of chickens lay different-color eggs. Most eggs are white or brown, but you can sometimes find pink, blue, or green eggs at the farmers' market. The color of the shell doesn't affect the egg's taste or texture.

When purchasing eggs, either at a grocery store or farmers' market, they should be refrigerated. Be sure to check the "sell-by" date to ensure freshness, and always inspect the eggs in the carton for cracks. Eggs should last for 3 to 5 weeks in the refrigerator.

Organic eggs do not contain antibiotics or hormones, and the hens that laid them ate organic feed. Studies have shown that these eggs have more omega-3 fatty acids and vitamins A and E than conventional eggs.

Prepping Poultry

Poultry requires a bit of care to prevent contamination and cross contamination. If you're thawing frozen poultry, place the package on a rimmed baking sheet or another vessel with an edge, and allow it to thaw in the refrigerator. Thawing poultry at room temperature can promote bacteria growth. Marinate poultry in the refrigerator as well

When you're ready to cook poultry, remove it from the package and place it on a clean cutting board. Trim excess fat from the meat and cut it down to the portion size you need. If you're preparing a whole chicken or turkey, remove the giblets from the cavity and any excess fat and pinfeathers from the skin. When prepping poultry, it's important to use a separate cutting board and knife to prevent cross contamination with other foods. I recommend prepping poultry last, when possible. As soon as you've finished handling the poultry, make sure you thoroughly wash your hands with soap and warm water for at least 20 seconds. Also, be sure to wipe down your prep area with soap and water.

How to Make an Omelet

Making a perfect omelet is a cooking technique that every home cook should master. There are many types of omelets, such as French, Spanish, Japanese, and diner-style. Italian frittatas are also a type of omelet. Once you master the basics, you can get creative, and you'll find that omelets are completely customizable. You'll be able to host a brunch with your very own omelet station.

BEST PRACTICES

When making an omelet, it's best to use a nonstick skillet. Even when using a nonstick skillet, you should still add butter so you create a surface where the eggs will not stick. The key is to keep the eggs moving and keep them from sticking to the pan. This is not the time to walk away from the stove.

To get started, whisk the eggs until they turn pale yellow and all the whites and yolks are fully incorporated. Preheat a 10-inch skillet over medium-low heat before adding the butter. Make sure the skillet is not too hot. If the butter sizzles when you add it, turn the heat down a bit. Once the butter has melted, add the egg mixture to the skillet, and allow it to sit for 1 minute, or until the bottom starts to set up. Use a rubber spatula to gently push the egg mixture a few inches toward the center of the skillet. Tilt the pan slightly to allow the liquid egg to run into the bare skillet. Continue this process until no more liquid egg mixture remains.

If you're planning to add fillings like meat, veggies, or cheese, prepare/cook them before cooking the eggs. Add up to a ½ cup on one-half of the egg. Using the spatula, fold the half without filling on top of the filling, then remove the omelet from the pan.

TROUBLESHOOTING MISTAKES

Making a perfect omelet can take practice. But that's okay, because even if your omelet doesn't look perfect, chances are it will still taste great.

If you find a piece of shell in the cracked eggs, use one of the eggshell halves to remove the errant shard. If you try to use your fingers or a spoon, you'll end up chasing the shell around the bowl and won't be able to get it.

Another common omelet mistake is adding too much filling. Overstuffing an omelet will cause it to break when it's folded. If you have too much filling, place the extras on top of the finished omelet.

How to Pound Chicken Cutlets

Many recipes using boneless, skinless chicken breast require you to pound the meat into thin cutlets because chicken breasts are not the same thickness throughout and can cook unevenly. The thinner end dries out, and the thick end is undercooked. Pounding the breast meat into a cutlet is an easy solution to ensure that the chicken is the same thickness throughout. It also helps tenderize the meat, and thinner pieces of chicken cook faster.

BEST PRACTICES

Start by placing one boneless, skinless chicken breast into a gallon-size zip-top bag. Remove as much air as possible, and seal it. Next, use a heavy object, such as a meat mallet, rolling pin, or canned good, and pound the chicken until the meat is an even thickness (about ½ inch) throughout. Remove the cutlet from the bag, and repeat the process with the remaining chicken. When pounding, always start at the thickest part of the chicken, and work your way toward the thinner end.

TROUBLESHOOTING MISTAKES

Be careful not to pound too hard; you don't want to break the chicken apart. If you don't have a zip-top bag, you can use two pieces of plastic wrap to pound chicken cutlets. Make sure the pieces of plastic wrap are triple the size of the chicken breast. Place the chicken breast between the two sheets of plastic and begin pounding, but do it more gently because the plastic wrap is thin.

How to Carve a Whole Turkey or Chicken

Whether you've cooked your own roast chicken (see Perfect Roast Chicken, page 86) or turkey or purchased a rotisserie chicken from the grocery store, knowing how to carve the bird is essential (and easy). I learned how to carve poultry by practicing on chickens. They are smaller and easier to handle than turkeys. Once you get the process down, you can take the skill on the road and tackle any size bird.

BEST PRACTICES

When carving chicken or turkey, it's important to have the right tools. A sharp knife is essential, as is a large cutting board. I prefer to use a cutting board with a groove along the edges to catch any juices that run out. The meat will be hot, so it helps to use a carving fork or even a dinner fork to hold the bird as you carve. Have paper towels or a kitchen towel handy to wipe your fingers, which will get slippery from the juice.

Tilt the cooked bird to remove any juices accumulated in the cavity, then place the bird, breast-side up with the legs toward you, on a large cutting board. Using a sharp carving or chef's knife, cut between the leg and the body to create a gap. This should expose the joint. Sever the joint with the knife, and remove the drumstick and thigh in one piece. You can then cut them apart by cutting down along the curve of the drumstick until you reach the joint. Cut through the joint to separate the two pieces. Repeat this process on the other leg.

Next, place the knife at the base of one side of the breast, above the wing. Make a cut starting at the wing and continuing until you reach the spot where the leg was. Use the knife to make a deep cut down along the breastbone on the top of the bird. The cut should be angled toward the first cut you made along the bottom of the breast. This should release one breast from the bone. Slice the breast meat into portions. Repeat this process on the other breast. The last step is to pull the wing away from the carcass and cut through the joint. Repeat this step on the other wing.

TROUBLESHOOTING MISTAKES

Keep in mind that carving won't change the flavor of the meat, only the presentation. Practice makes perfect.

One of the biggest mistakes when carving poultry is not letting the meat rest before cutting. Chicken needs to rest for at least 10 minutes and turkey for 20 minutes after cooking before you cut into it to allow the juices to redistribute into the meat.

Another common mistake is using the wrong knife. Use a carving knife or a 10-inch chef's knife to carve a bird; a smaller knife will lead to frustration.

Chicken Cutlets with Lemony Pan Sauce

Serves 4	**Prep time:** 10 minutes	**Cook time:** 25 minutes

Skills used: Pounding chicken cutlets, panfrying, measuring

1 cup all-purpose flour

1½ pounds or 4 (6-ounce) boneless, skinless chicken breasts, pounded into ½-inch-thick cutlets

2 teaspoons table salt, divided

½ teaspoon freshly ground black pepper, divided

2 tablespoons extra-virgin olive oil

3 tablespoons unsalted butter, divided

½ cup dry white wine (see Simple Rice Pilaf, Ingredient Tip, page 39)

1 lemon

½ cup low-sodium chicken broth

¼ cup chopped fresh parsley leaves

Per Serving: Calories: 412; Fat: 18g; Saturated fat: 7g; Cholesterol: 122mg; Carbohydrates: 13g; Fiber: 1g; Protein: 41g; Sodium: 1,071mg

This recipe will help you master the art of a simple pan sauce. Pan sauces are flavorful, customizable, and convenient because they are made in the same pan used to cook the meat and/or vegetables. The flavor comes from the fond, or bits of food stuck to the bottom of the pan. Liquid, such as stock, broth, citrus juice, or wine, deglazes or lifts the bits from the bottom of the pan to flavor the sauce.

1. Preheat the oven to 200°F.
2. Place the flour in a shallow bowl, such as a pie dish. Pat the pounded chicken cutlets dry with paper towels, and season with 1 teaspoon salt and ¼ teaspoon pepper.
3. In a large skillet, heat the olive oil and 2 tablespoons of butter over medium-high heat. When the butter has melted, place one chicken cutlet in the flour, and coat it on both sides. Shake off any excess flour, and place the cutlet in the skillet. Repeat with another piece of chicken, working in batches if needed.
4. Cook each cutlet for 3 to 4 minutes, or until the bottom is golden brown, then flip the chicken. Cook on the other side for 3 to 4 minutes or until that side is golden brown. Place all the cooked chicken on a rimmed baking sheet, and transfer it to the oven to keep warm.

5. Add wine to the same skillet, and scrape the bottom of the pan to loosen any bits of chicken. Simmer for 1 to 2 minutes, or until the wine has reduced by half.

6. While the wine is reducing, cut the lemon in half and squeeze the juice into a small bowl. Remove any seeds. Slice the juiced lemon into thin slices.

7. To the skillet with the wine, now add the lemon juice, lemon slices, chicken broth, 1 teaspoon salt, and the remaining ¼ teaspoon pepper. Simmer for 2 to 3 minutes or until the sauce has reduced and started to thicken slightly. Stir in the remaining 1 tablespoon butter, and whisk until melted.

8. Add the chicken and any juices that accumulated on the baking sheet back into the skillet, and simmer for 3 to 4 minutes or until the chicken reaches 165°F on a meat thermometer. To serve the chicken, transfer it to a serving platter, and spoon the sauce over top. Garnish with lemon slices from the pan and chopped parsley.

9. To store leftovers, allow the dish to cool completely, place it in a container with a tight-fitting lid, and refrigerate for up to 4 days.

INGREDIENT TIP: When pounding chicken cutlets, it's important to get them to approximately the same thickness, so that they cook evenly (see How to Pound Chicken Cutlets, page 77).

Soothing Chicken Noodle Soup

Serves 4	**Prep time:** 20 minutes	**Cook time:** 40 minutes

Skills used: Knife skills, measuring

1 tablespoon unsalted butter
1 carrot, diced
1 celery stalk, diced
½ yellow onion, diced
2 garlic cloves, minced
4 cups low-sodium chicken stock
1 whole bay leaf
1 teaspoon table salt
¼ teaspoon freshly ground black pepper
1½ pounds bone-in, skin-on chicken breasts
1 cup wide egg noodles
1 tablespoon chopped fresh parsley leaves
1 tablespoon chopped fresh dill

Per Serving: Calories: 273; Fat: 14g; Saturated fat: 5g; Cholesterol: 88mg; Carbohydrates: 10g; Fiber: 1g; Protein: 26g; Sodium: 675mg

Now when your friends are sick, you, too, can come calling with your very own homemade chicken soup. This comforting recipe is easy to double so you can freeze some for a later date. If you do freeze the soup, make it without the noodles. If you store the noodles in the soup, they will continue to absorb the liquid and become mushy. When you're ready to reheat the soup, just add the noodles and simmer until tender.

1. In a large stockpot or Dutch oven, melt the butter over medium heat.

2. Add the carrot, celery, and onion. Cook, stirring occasionally, until tender, 3 to 4 minutes. Stir in the garlic, and cook until fragrant, about 1 minute. Pour in the chicken stock, and add the bay leaf, salt, and pepper.

3. Remove the skin from the chicken breasts by running your fingers underneath and pulling it off, discard the skin, add the chicken (still on the bone) to the pot, and bring it to a boil. Once boiling, reduce the heat, cover the pot with a lid, and simmer for 30 minutes or until the chicken reaches an internal temperature of 165° on a meat thermometer.

4. Remove the chicken breasts from the pot, and use a fork to pull the meat from the bones. Add the shredded chicken back to the pot, and stir in the noodles. Simmer for 6 to 7 minutes or until the noodles are tender. Remove the pot from the heat, remove the bay leaf, stir in the chopped parsley and dill, and add more salt and pepper to taste.

5. To store leftovers, allow the soup to cool completely, place it in a container with a tight-fitting lid, and refrigerate for up to 4 days.

INGREDIENT TIP: If you prefer dark meat (less heart-healthy but more flavorful), you can use an equal amount of bone-in, skinless chicken thighs in this recipe.

Sheet-Pan Chicken Shawarma

Serves 4	**Prep time:** 10 minutes	**Cook time:** 20 minutes

Skills used: Slicing, measuring

Shawarma is a popular Turkish street food combining warm chicken or meat, warm spices, and warm pita. The name comes from the technique traditionally used to make the dish—shawarma (translated as "turning" in Arabic) entails cooking meat by stacking it and then turning it on a vertical rotisserie. Here, we won't truly shawarma the shawarma but will bake it instead, using spices reminiscent of the authentic dish. To serve, pile the chicken on a warmed pita, and add chopped cucumber and tomatoes. Drizzle the tahini sauce on top.

FOR THE CHICKEN
- 1 cup plain Greek yogurt
- 2 tablespoons shawarma seasoning blend (see Ingredient Tip)
- 1½ pounds boneless, skinless chicken breasts, sliced against the grain into 1-inch strips
- 1 tablespoon extra-virgin olive oil
- 2 red bell peppers, seeded and cut into ½-inch strips
- 1 red onion, cut into ½-inch pieces
- ½ cup pimentos
- 4 pitas, warmed

FOR THE SAUCE
- 1 cup tahini
- 4 garlic cloves, minced
- ⅔ cup water
- ½ cup freshly squeezed lemon juice, from 2½ lemons
- ⅓ cup extra-virgin olive oil
- ½ teaspoon table salt

Per Serving: Calories: 532; Fat: 26g; Saturated fat: 5g; Cholesterol: 132mg; Carbohydrates: 29g; Fiber: 6g; Protein: 47g; Sodium: 399mg

1. Preheat the oven to 350°F.
2. **To make the chicken:** In a large bowl, stir together the Greek yogurt and shawarma seasoning blend. Add the chicken strips to the yogurt mixture and stir until the chicken is completely coated; set it aside.
3. Drizzle the olive oil on a rimmed baking sheet, and arrange the coated chicken (discard any marinade that remains in the bowl), bell peppers, onion, and pimentos in an even layer.

4. Bake for 20 minutes or until the internal temperature of the chicken is 165°F on a meat thermometer.

5. **To make the sauce:** While the chicken is baking, in a medium bowl, whisk together the tahini, garlic, water, lemon juice, olive oil, and salt until it's smooth.

6. Pile the chicken into split, warmed pitas, and top it with the sauce, and with chopped cucumber and tomato, if you'd like.

7. To store leftovers, allow the chicken to cool completely, place it in a container with a tight-fitting lid, and refrigerate for up to 4 days.

INGREDIENT TIP: If you can't find shawarma seasoning, you can easily make your own. Combine 2 teaspoons each of cumin, cardamom, turmeric, cinnamon, and salt in a small bowl and stir.

Perfect Roast Chicken

Serves 4	**Prep time:** 10 minutes, plus 20 minutes to rest	**Cook time:** 1 hour 35 minutes

Skills used: Knife skills, measuring, roasting

1 (4- to 5-pound) whole roasting chicken (or see Variation Tip)

3½ teaspoons table salt, divided

½ teaspoon freshly ground black pepper, divided

1 large bunch fresh thyme, plus 20 sprigs, divided

1 lemon, halved

1 garlic head, halved crosswise

2 tablespoons unsalted butter, melted

Kitchen string

1 large yellow onion, cut into 8 wedges

4 carrots, cut into chunks

2 celery stalks (leave the tops on), cut into chunks

Per Serving: Calories: 546; Fat: 37g; Saturated fat: 13g; Cholesterol: 171mg; Carbohydrates: 11g; Fiber: 3g; Protein: 40g; Sodium: 787mg

Learning how to make a whole roast chicken is a great skill for a beginner cook and is an especially effective way to serve (and impress) a crowd. The process is fairly simple, and the finished chicken is a showstopper. You can use the leftovers in all sorts of things, such as casseroles, soups, sandwiches, and salads. Serve it with Mashed Potatoes in a Snap (page 52) and/or Robust Roasted Root Vegetables (page 53) and you'll have a hearty and wholesome meal.

1. Preheat the oven to 350°F.

2. Remove the chicken giblets from the cavity, remove any excess fat and pinfeathers from the skin, and pat dry with paper towels.

3. Season the inside cavity of the chicken with half of the salt and pepper. Stuff the cavity with the bunch of thyme, both lemon halves, and both garlic halves. Brush the outside of the chicken with melted butter, and season it with the other half of the salt and ground black pepper.

4. Use kitchen string to tie the legs together, then tuck the wing tips under the chicken body. In the bottom of a roasting pan, place the onion, carrots, and celery, along with the 20 sprigs of thyme.

5. Set the chicken on top of the vegetables, and roast for 20 minutes per pound of chicken, plus an extra 15 minutes. A 4-pound chicken would roast for 1 hour, 35 minutes. The chicken is done when the internal temperature reaches 165°F on a meat thermometer inserted between the leg and breast. If you notice that the skin of the chicken is getting too brown as it cooks, cover it loosely with a piece of aluminum foil. This protects the skin as the chicken continues to cook.

6. Remove the chicken from the oven and cover it with foil; allow it to rest for 15 minutes before carving (see How to Carve a Whole Turkey or Chicken, page 78).

7. To store leftovers, allow the chicken to cool completely, carve the chicken, and place pieces in a container with a tight-fitting lid. Refrigerate for up to 4 days.

VARIATION TIP: The same recipe and process can be used to roast a whole turkey. Increase the amount of butter to ½ cup (1 stick). Roast the turkey for 13 minutes per pound of turkey and allow it to rest for 20 minutes before carving.

Denver Omelet

| Serves 1 | **Prep time:** 10 minutes | **Cook time:** 5 minutes |

Skills used: Knife skills, measuring, dicing, sautéing

3 large eggs
⅛ teaspoon table salt
⅛ teaspoon freshly ground black pepper
2 tablespoons unsalted butter, divided
¼ cup diced thick-cut smoked ham
¼ cup diced red onion
2 tablespoons diced bell pepper
2 tablespoons shredded cheddar cheese

Per Serving: Calories: 543; Fat: 45g; Saturated fat: 23g; Cholesterol: 649mg; Carbohydrates: 7g; Fiber: 1g; Protein: 28g; Sodium: 748mg

This Denver omelet, also known as the western omelet, is a diner classic filled with ham, onion, bell peppers, and cheese. It's a quick meal to make, but you can speed it up even more by using frozen diced peppers and onions in place of fresh ones. Thaw the frozen vegetables and drain off any excess liquid before adding them to the skillet. Plus, omelet fillings can be tailored specifically to your liking. Don't like meat? Add more veggies. Love meat? Add some bacon.

1. In a medium bowl, crack the eggs. Add the salt and pepper, and whisk until there are no streaks of white or yellow. Set them aside.

2. Heat a 10-inch nonstick skillet over medium heat, and melt 1 tablespoon of butter. When the butter has melted, add the ham, and sauté for 1 to 2 minutes or until lightly browned. Add the diced onion and diced bell pepper, and sauté for about 2 minutes or until the vegetables are crisp-tender. Transfer the ham and vegetables to a plate, and wipe out the skillet with paper towels.

3. Return the skillet to the stove, adjust the heat to medium-low, and melt the remaining 1 tablespoon butter.

4. When the butter has melted, add the eggs to the skillet, and allow them to sit for 1 minute or until the bottom of the eggs start to set. Using a rubber spatula, gently push the egg mixture a few inches toward the center of the skillet, and tilt the pan slightly, allowing the liquid egg from the top to run into the bare skillet. Continue this process until no more liquid egg mixture remains (see How to Make an Omelet, page 76).

5. Turn the heat off, and add the cooked ham, onions, and peppers on top of one half of the omelet. Top with the shredded cheese, and use the spatula to flip the empty half of the omelet on top of the filling. Carefully, use the spatula to slide the omelet out of the pan and onto a plate.

6. To store leftovers, allow the omelet to cool completely, place it in a container with a tight-fitting lid, and refrigerate for up to 2 days.

SUBSTITUTION TIP: If you want to make a healthier omelet, use egg whites instead (and replace the ham with extra veggies). One whole egg equals the whites from 2 eggs. Or if you have a carton of egg whites, 3 tablespoons plus 2 teaspoons replace 1 large egg.

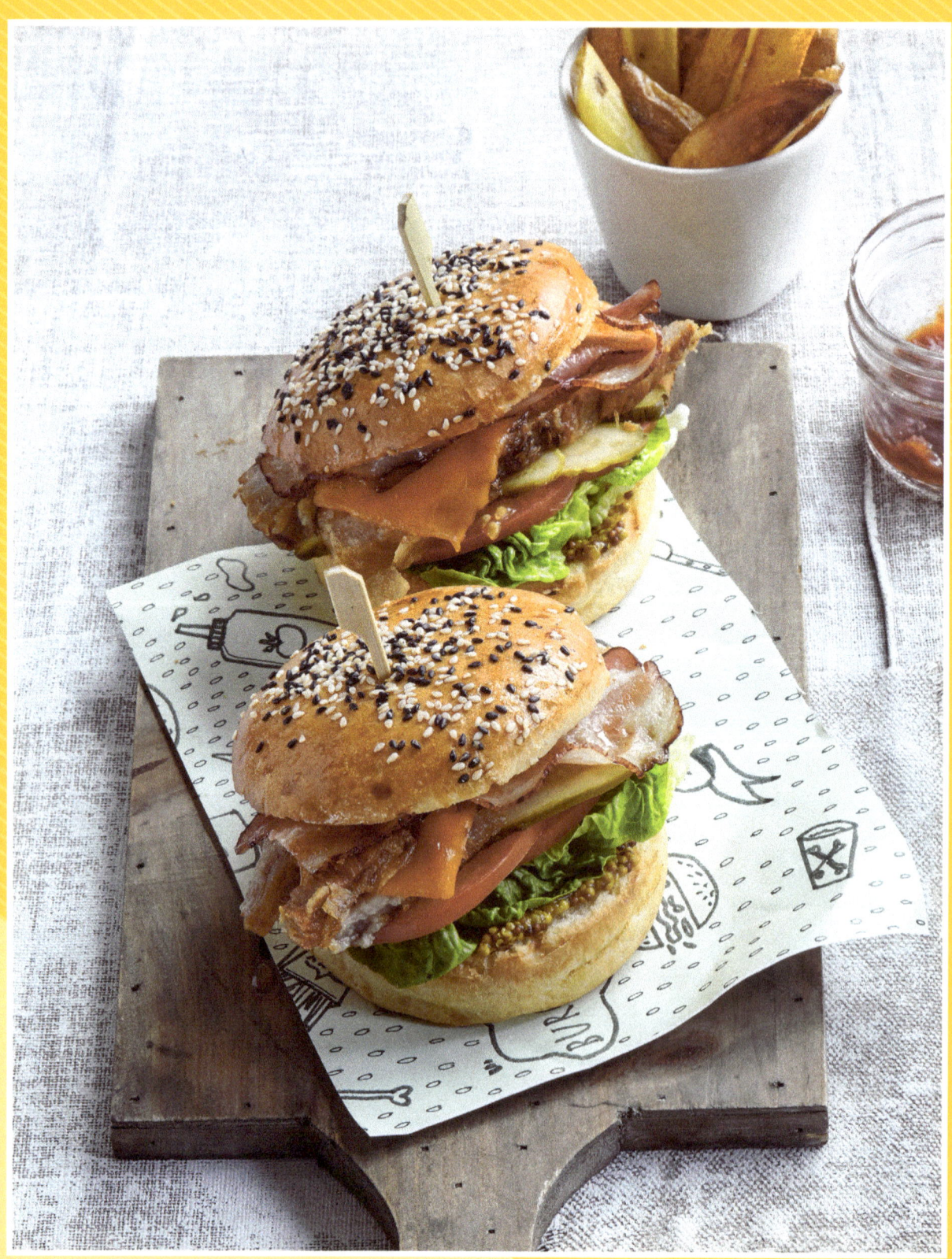

Grilled Bacon Cheeseburger, page 98.

CHAPTER 7

Beef, Pork, and Lamb

Beef, pork, and lamb are the most common red meats. In this chapter, you'll learn about how to purchase quality meat. You'll also learn some basic preparations and essential techniques, such as how to slice meat against the grain, how to cook bacon perfectly, and how to cook and drain ground beef.

Grilled Bacon Cheeseburger 98

Easy-Breezy Beef Tacos 100

Apricot Miso Pork Tenderloin 102

Skillet Pork Chops with Mustard Pan Sauce 104

Garlic and Herb Lamb Chops 106

Meet Your Meat

Meat is categorized into two varieties: white, which includes poultry; and red, which includes beef, pork, and lamb. Red meats are protein-rich and contain a variety of vitamins and minerals that our bodies require. Of the three types of red meat, beef has the highest fat percentage.

One of the easiest ways to tell the difference between these meats is their color. They are all considered red meats, but beef has the darkest red color of the three. Lamb is also quite red in coloring. Pork is the lightest in color of the three types.

Generally, the leanest and most tender cuts of beef, pork, and lamb come from the loin. These cuts come from areas that don't get much exercise, which keeps the muscle tender. The tougher cuts of these meats come from the shoulder, rump, and leg areas. These areas move a lot, so the muscles become tougher. When you look at meat, you will notice white ribbons of fat throughout. This is called marbling and is what makes meat tender, moist, and flavorful.

When it comes to taste, lamb and beef are very similar, but lamb tends to be more tender and has a more grassy, robust flavor. Pork is often referred to as white meat because the texture and flavor are closer to poultry than beef.

All of these meats are widely available in grocery stores. You can also purchase them from local butchers or farmers.

BEEF

When buying beef, you can learn a lot from the label. Each package should clearly state the cut, grade, weight, price per pound, and sell-by date. When selecting beef, you want to choose bright red meat that is firm to the touch.

The United States Department of Agriculture (USDA) grades the quality of retail beef into several categories: prime, choice, and select. Prime is the highest quality, most expensive, and has the most marbling, making the beef tender and juicy. Choice beef is the middle of the road, with less marbling but good flavor and texture. Select is the least expensive, has the least marbling, and has more fat. It is often sold under the store brand and needs more intervention to make it tender.

Steaks and tenderloins are the more expensive cuts of beef because they are so tender and because there are fewer of them per carcass. Chuck roast and round steaks are more affordable. These cuts usually require longer cooking times because they are tougher, but they contain lots of flavor. If you're looking for leaner cuts, look for the word "loin" in the cut.

Ground beef also has a range of quality and pricing based on fat percentage and type of beef (chuck, round, sirloin). Sirloin is priciest because it's a higher (steak level) quality and is also fairly lean. Round is the leanest and is the middle of the road. Chuck is the least expensive because it usually has more fat. But again, fat equals flavor, so chuck is more flavorful.

Beef should be used or frozen within two days of purchase. Color is not a good indicator of beef that has gone bad. If the meat is slimy, tacky, or has a strong odor, discard it.

Beef doneness can range from 120°F for rare to 160°F for well-done. According to the USDA, roasts and steaks should be cooked to a minimum of 145°F (which is medium; medium-well is 150°F), and ground beef should be cooked to 160°F. If you prefer to cook beef to a lower temperature/doneness (medium-rare is 135°F), do so with caution and at your own risk.

It's important to remember that meat will continue to cook when removed from the heat. Steaks and burgers should be taken off the heat when the internal temperature is 5°F lower than the desired temperature. Roasts should be removed when the internal temperature is between 5 and 10°F lower than the desired temperature.

LAMB

Lamb is widely available from grocery stores, butchers, and farmers. Packages are clearly labeled with the cut, grade, weight, price per pound, and sell-by date. When selecting lamb, choose pinkish-red meat with white marbling throughout.

Like beef, the USDA grades lamb into several retail categories—prime, choice, and good. The grade is dependent on quality factors such as leanness and color. Prime is the highest quality, and good meets lesser standards. Most grocers carry prime and choice cuts.

Chops and cutlets are the more expensive cuts of lamb. If you are looking for more affordable cuts, try the shoulder, neck, leg, or sirloin roast. Like beef, these cuts will require longer cooking times to become tender.

Raw ground lamb and stew meat cuts can be stored in the refrigerator for up to 2 days, and chops and roasts can be kept for up to 5 days. Similar to beef, you can easily recognize lamb that is not good by inspecting the smell and feel. A slimy or tacky feel indicates that meat is past its prime.

Like beef, the USDA recommends that whole cuts of lamb be cooked to a minimum of 145°F and ground lamb should be cooked to 160°F. Again, the meat will continue to cook when removed from the heat, so it's best to take it off when the internal temperature is between 5 and 10°F lower than the desired temperature.

PORK

The USDA does not grade pork like it does beef and lamb. Instead, color, marbling, water capacity, and pH measure pork quality. When shopping for pork, look for reddish-pink meat that is firm to the touch. The package should not have any excess liquid. You also want to look for some marbling throughout the meat. The package should also have a USDA stamp, indicating that it was inspected.

Pork tenderloin and pork loin chops are the most expensive cuts, and pork shoulder, spareribs, ground pork, and sirloin chops are more affordable. There are also cured pork products, such as bacon, ham, and sausages. Cured pork is preserved through smoking, salting, aging, drying, or brining. Relatively speaking, pork costs less than lamb or beef. Raw whole cuts can be stored in the refrigerator for up to 5 days, but ground pork should only be kept for up to 2 days.

The USDA recommends that whole cuts of pork be cooked to a minimum of 145°F and ground pork should be cooked to 160°F. Like beef and lamb, the meat will continue to cook after it is removed from the heat, so it's best to remove it when the internal temperature is between 5 and 10°F lower than the desired temperature.

Prepping Cuts

To prepare red meat for cooking, start by trimming away any excess fat. You don't need to remove all the fat from the meat, because fat adds flavor. Just remove any larger sections that won't render off when cooking. Once trimmed, pat the meat dry with a paper towel; excess moisture will prevent the meat from browning when cooking. Season meats liberally with salt and pepper to enhance their natural flavor.

Beef, lamb, and pork can be prepared in a number of ways, depending on the cut of meat. For more information on meat cuts, cooking tips, and recommendations, check out the Resources (page 146).

How to Slice Meat Against the Grain

The grain of the meat refers to the direction the muscle fibers run. The key to properly slicing meat is to identify the direction of the grain and slice across it, not parallel to it. Here's why: Animal muscle fibers are naturally tough because the animal uses them to move. By slicing the meat against the grain, you shorten the meat fibers, making it easier and more tender to chew.

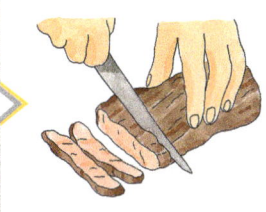

In some cuts, it's easier to find the grain than in others. The grain can also change directions, so you may have to shift the direction you're cutting. Every cut of meat is different, so it's important to assess the direction of the grain before cutting it.

BEST PRACTICES

When slicing meat, use a cutting board and a sharp knife. A chef's knife or carving knife works best. The knife's blade should be long enough to go through the meat in one slice.

To keep the cutting board from sliding around, place a damp paper towel underneath it. Grip the knife firmly, and use your other hand or a carving fork to hold the meat in place. If using your hand, be sure to tuck your fingertips under. After determining the direction of the grain, slice the meat in a single slice using the entire blade. Don't use a sawing motion as you go through.

The thickness of the whole piece of meat is something else you want to consider when you're slicing meat. Even if you slice thicker cuts of meat, such as beef brisket, against the grain, it can still be tough. In this case, you should try to slice the meat thinner to make it easier to chew.

TROUBLESHOOTING MISTAKES

If you find that you can't run the knife through the meat without sawing back and forth, you need to sharpen the knife.

Another common mistake is not letting the meat rest. You should always let meat sit for half the time it took to cook it. Allowing the meat to rest before cutting it gives the juices time to work back into the meat. If you cut into it without letting it rest, the juices will run out onto the cutting board, leaving you with a drier piece of meat.

How to Cook Bacon Perfectly

Cooking bacon on the stovetop can be a messy job. You can only fit a few slices in the pan at once, the slices don't always cook evenly, and bacon grease splatters all over the cooktop. There is an easier (and less messy) way to make perfect bacon: baking it.

BEST PRACTICES

Start by preheating the oven to 400°F. Line a rimmed baking sheet with aluminum foil to minimize cleanup and place the bacon slices in a single layer on the baking sheet, ensuring the slices do not overlap.

Place the bacon in the oven (it does not need to be fully preheated) and bake for 12 to 17 minutes, depending on the thickness of the bacon. Start checking doneness around 10 minutes. Look for your desired crispiness—the longer it bakes, the browner and crispier the bacon becomes. There is no need to flip the bacon.

Remove the cooked bacon from the baking sheet as soon as it comes out of the oven. Otherwise, the bacon will continue to cook. Transfer the bacon slices to a paper-towel-lined plate in a single layer using tongs or a fork. If you need to, add another layer of paper towels on top of the first layer of bacon, and continue to layer as needed. The paper towels will absorb some of the excess bacon fat.

TROUBLESHOOTING MISTAKES

The oven does not have to be fully preheated before adding the bacon. If it is preheated to 400°F, check the bacon for doneness sooner. As the bacon cooks, it will release fat, and the bacon will cook in the fat. Watch it because bacon will burn very quickly.

When the bacon is done cooking, don't pour the bacon fat down the drain. As the fat cools, it will solidify on the sides of the drain and can cause plumbing issues. Instead, allow the fat to cool in the pan, wrap up the foil, and toss it in the trash.

How to Cook and Drain Ground Beef

Ground beef is one of the most common types of meat available. It's flavorful, affordable, and can be used in many recipes for many different things. There are some basic techniques to follow to ensure that beef is cooked perfectly.

BEST PRACTICES

When cooking ground meat, choosing the right size skillet is essential. For 1 to 1½ pounds of ground meat, you should use a 10- or 12-inch skillet. This provides enough surface area for the meat to cook evenly. If the skillet is too small, the meat will steam and not brown properly. For cooking other quantities of meat, size the pan up or down accordingly.

The best way to get started is to pour oil (canola, olive, or vegetable) into a skillet and heat it over medium-high heat. When the oil is shimmering and the skillet is hot, you add the beef. Season it with salt and pepper to taste, and use a spatula or wooden spoon to break the meat up into smaller pieces as soon as you add it to the skillet. This will help the meat brown more evenly. As the beef cooks, continue breaking it up into smaller pieces but try not to move it around too much. You want to give it enough time to brown.

When the meat is cooked through, it will be uniformly browned with no pink remaining, and will read 160°F on a meat thermometer. Turn off the heat. To drain the excess fat from the meat, use a spatula or spoon to push the meat to one side of the pan and tilt it, allowing the fat to pool in the open area. Keeping the pan tilted, use a spoon to remove as much fat as possible, and put the fat in a bowl. When most of the fat has been removed, you can use a wad of paper towels to absorb the remaining fat from the pooled area (watch your fingers!).

You can use the same process for cooking ground pork, lamb, chicken, or turkey.

TROUBLESHOOTING MISTAKES

Like bacon fat, the fat from ground meat should not be poured down the sink drain. The cooled fat will cling to the pipes and can cause plumbing issues. Allow the fat to cool in the bowl and, when it has solidified, scrape it into the trash.

Grilled Bacon Cheeseburger

Serves 4	**Prep time:** 10 minutes, plus 5 minutes to rest	**Cook time:** 8 minutes

Skills used: Measuring, grilling

1⅓ pounds ground beef
2 teaspoons table salt
2 teaspoons freshly ground black pepper
2 teaspoons onion powder
2 teaspoons garlic powder
4 slices cheddar cheese
4 burger buns
8 slices cooked bacon (see How to Cook Bacon Perfectly, page 96)

Per Serving: Calories: 672; Fat: 42g; Saturated fat: 17g; Cholesterol: 154mg; Carbohydrates: 24g; Fiber: 1g; Protein: 47g; Sodium: 1,765mg

No more fast food for you (although this recipe is pretty fast). Make a homemade version of this classic comfort food. Ground beef is sold according to the amount of lean meat to fat. You can use any type of ground beef for this recipe, such as 80/20 or 90/10 blends. Keep in mind, though, that leaner blends will produce less-juicy burgers. I often use an 80/20 blend because the extra fat adds more flavor.

1. Preheat the grill (see Preparation Tip for stovetop method) to medium-high.

2. In a large bowl, combine the beef, salt, pepper, onion powder, and garlic powder. Gently mix with your hands until just combined. Be careful not to overmix.

3. Divide the seasoned meat into four equal portions, and form into patties. Using your thumb, make an indent about the size of a quarter in the center of each patty, so that the burger patties do not puff in the center when cooked.

4. Place the burgers on the grill over medium-high heat for about 3 minutes per side for medium-rare (135°F on a meat thermometer) or 4 to 5 minutes per side to reach the USDA-recommended temperature of 160°F. During the last 2 minutes of grilling, place one cheese slice on top of each burger. Turn off the heat, and transfer the burgers to a plate. Cover the plate with aluminum foil, and allow the burgers to rest for 5 minutes.

5. Place the cheeseburgers on the bottom halves of the buns, and top each cheeseburger with two slices of cooked bacon. Top with the other half of the bun.

6. To store leftovers, allow the burgers to cool completely, place them in a container with a tight-fitting lid, and refrigerate for up to 4 days.

FLAVOR BOOST: For a Southwestern twist on this recipe, in step 2, replace the seasonings with 3 teaspoons of taco seasoning. Grill the burgers as directed and, in step 4, replace the cheddar cheese with pepper Jack cheese. Top with Classic Guacamole (page 130).

PREPARATION TIP: These burgers can also be prepared on the stovetop. In step 1, preheat a large cast-iron skillet over medium-high heat. Prepare the burgers and then put 1 tablespoon of butter in the skillet. Once the butter has melted, place the prepared burger patties in the preheated skillet and cook as directed.

Easy-Breezy Beef Tacos

Serves 4	**Prep time:** 5 minutes	**Cook time:** 15 minutes

Skills used: Measuring, draining ground beef

1 pound ground beef
1 tablespoon chili powder
¾ teaspoon ground cumin
½ teaspoon table salt
½ teaspoon dried oregano
½ teaspoon garlic powder
¼ teaspoon onion powder
½ cup canned tomato sauce
8 taco shells

Per Serving: Calories: 337; Fat: 17g; Saturated fat: 6g; Cholesterol: 74mg; Carbohydrates: 19g; Fiber: 3g; Protein: 25g; Sodium: 510mg

Now you, too, can participate in Taco Tuesdays with this straightforward but delicious recipe. This beefy taco filling is seasoned with a homemade taco seasoning and cooked in a rich tomato sauce to give it a unique flair. If you have leftovers, you can add it to the No-Sweat Three-Bean Chili (page 34) for extra protein. Use whatever taco toppings your heart desires, from lettuce to shredded cheese, salsa to Classic Guacamole (page 130).

1. Heat a large skillet over medium heat. Put the ground beef in the heated skillet, and break it up with a spoon or spatula into small pieces as it cooks. Add the chili powder, cumin, salt, oregano, garlic powder, and onion powder to the beef. Cook about it for 8 to 10 minutes until browned and no longer pink.

2. Drain any excess fat from the skillet (see How to Cook and Drain Ground Beef, page 97) and return the skillet to the stove.

3. Reduce the heat to low, and pour the tomato sauce in the skillet with the drained ground beef. Stir until the meat is completely coated in the sauce, and simmer for 5 minutes. The sauce will thicken slightly.

4. Fill the taco shells with the beef mixture, and add your favorite toppings.

5. To store leftovers, allow the beef to cool completely, place it in a container with a tight-fitting lid, and refrigerate for up to 4 days.

SUBSTITUTION TIP: For a lighter, leaner taco, replace the ground beef with ground turkey, chicken, or pork.

Apricot Miso Pork Tenderloin

Serves 4	**Prep time:** 10 minutes, plus 8 minutes to rest	**Cook time:** 35 minutes

Skills used: Knife skills, measuring, mincing, roasting, slicing meat

Nonstick cooking spray

¼ cup plus 1 tablespoon apricot preserves

¼ cup white miso (see Ingredient Tip)

¼ cup rice wine vinegar

1 large garlic clove, minced

2 (1-pound) pork tenderloins

¾ teaspoon table salt, divided

¼ teaspoon plus ⅛ teaspoon freshly ground black pepper, divided

½ cup low-sodium chicken broth

Per Serving: Calories: 371; Fat: 9g; Saturated fat: 3g; Cholesterol: 147mg; Carbohydrates: 21g; Fiber: 1g; Protein: 49g; Sodium: 1,207mg

Talk about a recipe to impress your guests. This recipe is the perfect combination of tangy, sweet, salty, and umami all at once. Keep in mind that pork tenderloin is a fairly lean cut, so it can overcook quickly. Closely monitor the temperature of the pork toward the end of the cooking time so that it doesn't dry out. Allowing the meat to rest before slicing it helps the pork stay tender and juicy.

1. Preheat the oven to 425°F. Coat a large, rimmed baking sheet with the cooking spray.

2. In a small pot, heat the apricot preserves, miso, vinegar, and garlic over medium. Cook for 1 to 2 minutes, until the mixture thickens slightly. Remove it from the heat, and set aside.

3. Pat the pork dry. Season both sides of each pork tenderloin with ½ teaspoon salt and ¼ teaspoon pepper. Place the tenderloins on the prepared baking sheet so they are not touching. Brush each tenderloin with 1 tablespoon apricot glaze.

4. Roast for 15 minutes; turn tenderloins over, and brush each tenderloin with 2 more tablespoons of apricot glaze.

5. Roast for an additional 10 minutes, or until the internal temperature of the pork reaches 140°F on a meat thermometer. Remove the pork from the oven, and allow it to rest on the baking sheet for 6 to 8 minutes.

6. While the pork is resting, in the pot with the remaining apricot glaze, add the chicken broth, remaining ¼ teaspoon salt, and ⅛ teaspoon pepper, and simmer over medium-high heat for 5 minutes or until the liquid has reduced, and the sauce has thickened slightly.

7. Slice the pork crosswise (see How to Slice Meat Against the Grain, page 95) into ½-inch-thick slices and spoon the sauce over the top.

8. To store leftovers, allow the tenderloins to cool completely, place them in a container with a tight-fitting lid, and refrigerate for up to 4 days.

INGREDIENT TIP: Miso is made from fermented soybeans. It has a savory, salty-sweet flavor. There are three types of miso: white, yellow, and red. White miso has the mildest flavor, and red is the strongest. If you're feeling adventurous, try using red miso in this recipe.

Skillet Pork Chops with Mustard Pan Sauce

Serves 4	**Prep time:** 5 minutes	**Cook time:** 15 minutes

Skills used: Measuring, sautéing

4 boneless pork chops, about ½-inch thick (see Ingredient Tip)
1½ teaspoons table salt, divided
1 tablespoon all-purpose flour
1 teaspoon chili powder
1 teaspoon garlic powder
1 teaspoon onion powder
1 tablespoon extra-virgin olive oil
½ cup low-sodium chicken broth
1 tablespoon freshly squeezed lemon juice
1 tablespoon Dijon mustard
¼ teaspoon Worcestershire sauce
1 tablespoon unsalted butter

Per Serving: Calories: 216; Fat: 10g; Saturated fat: 4g; Cholesterol: 82mg; Carbohydrates: 3g; Fiber: 1g; Protein: 26g; Sodium: 995mg

These tender pork chops are cooked with a bright and tangy pan sauce, a technique I also discuss in the poultry chapter because it's so versatile. The liquid deglazes the pan so it releases any flavorful bits of meat stuck to the bottom. The result is a sauce that's full of flavor and perfectly pairs with the meat you're cooking. Serve these on top of Mashed Potatoes in a Snap (page 52) or with some crusty bread.

1. Season all sides of the pork chops with 1 teaspoon salt, and set aside.

2. In a small bowl, combine the flour, chili powder, garlic powder, and onion powder. Stir to combine. Coat both sides of the pork chops in the spice rub.

3. In a skillet, heat the olive oil over medium-high heat. When the oil is shimmery and the pan is hot, add the pork chops. Cook the pork chops for 2 to 3 minutes or until the bottom is golden brown. Flip the chops, and cook for 3 to 4 minutes longer or until the pork reaches 145°F on a meat thermometer. Transfer the pork chops to a dish, and cover with foil.

4. Place the same skillet back on the stove over medium-high heat. In the skillet, combine the chicken broth, lemon juice, mustard, Worcestershire sauce, and remaining ½ teaspoon salt, stirring to loosen any bits from the bottom of the skillet. Bring the sauce to a simmer, and cook until the sauce has thickened, 4 to 5 minutes.

5. Remove the skillet from the heat, and stir in the butter. Add the pork chops back into the skillet, and reheat for 2 to 3 minutes. Serve the pork chops with sauce drizzled over top.

6. To store leftovers, allow the pork chops to cool completely, place them in a container with a tight-fitting lid, and refrigerate for up to 4 days.

INGREDIENT TIP: They sell thin-cut pork chops in most grocery stores. If you can't find them, cut thicker 1-inch pork chops in half.

VARIATION TIP: The sauce in this recipe goes great with pork or chicken. You can easily substitute boneless, skinless chicken cutlets for the pork chops.

Garlic and Herb Lamb Chops

Serves 4	**Prep time:** 10 minutes, plus 1 hour to marinate and 7 minutes to rest	**Cook time:** 12 minutes

Skills used: Knife skills, measuring, chopping, mincing

8 lamb loin chops
1½ teaspoons table salt
½ teaspoon freshly ground black pepper
2 tablespoons minced garlic
1 tablespoon extra-virgin olive oil
1 tablespoon chopped fresh rosemary
1 tablespoon chopped fresh thyme
1 teaspoon chopped fresh parsley
2 tablespoons unsalted butter

Per Serving: Calories: 426; Fat: 39g; Saturated fat: 17g; Cholesterol: 94mg; Carbohydrates: 2g; Fiber: 0g; Protein: 18g; Sodium: 945mg

Lamb chops might seem like something you order at a fancy restaurant, but I promise you, they're even better (and much cheaper) when you make them at home. When you see how quick, easy, and mouthwatering these are, you'll become a huge fan. This recipe uses loin chops, which are leaner and more tender than rib chops. These lamb chops get their flavor from a garlic and herb paste. The chops need to marinate for at least 1 hour but can sit for up to 8 hours, covered in the refrigerator.

1. Season both sides of the lamb chops with the salt and pepper.

2. In a small bowl, combine the garlic, olive oil, rosemary, thyme, and parsley until it's a paste. Divide the paste evenly among the chops, and rub it over both sides of each chop.

3. Place the chops in a container, cover, and refrigerate for at least 1 hour or up to 8 hours.

4. In a large skillet, heat the butter over medium-high heat. When the butter has melted, add the marinated lamb chops, and cook for 2 to 3 minutes or until the bottom is golden brown. Flip the chops, and (for medium-well) cook for 5 to 6 minutes or until the internal temperature is 145°F on a meat thermometer. Allow the lamb chops to rest for 5 to 7 minutes before serving.

5. To store leftovers, allow the chops to cool completely, place them in a container with a tight-fitting lid, and refrigerate for up to 3 days.

INGREDIENT TIP: The USDA recommends cooking lamb to an internal temperature of 145°F (medium-well). When lamb is cooked beyond this point, it can become tough and take on a gamy flavor.

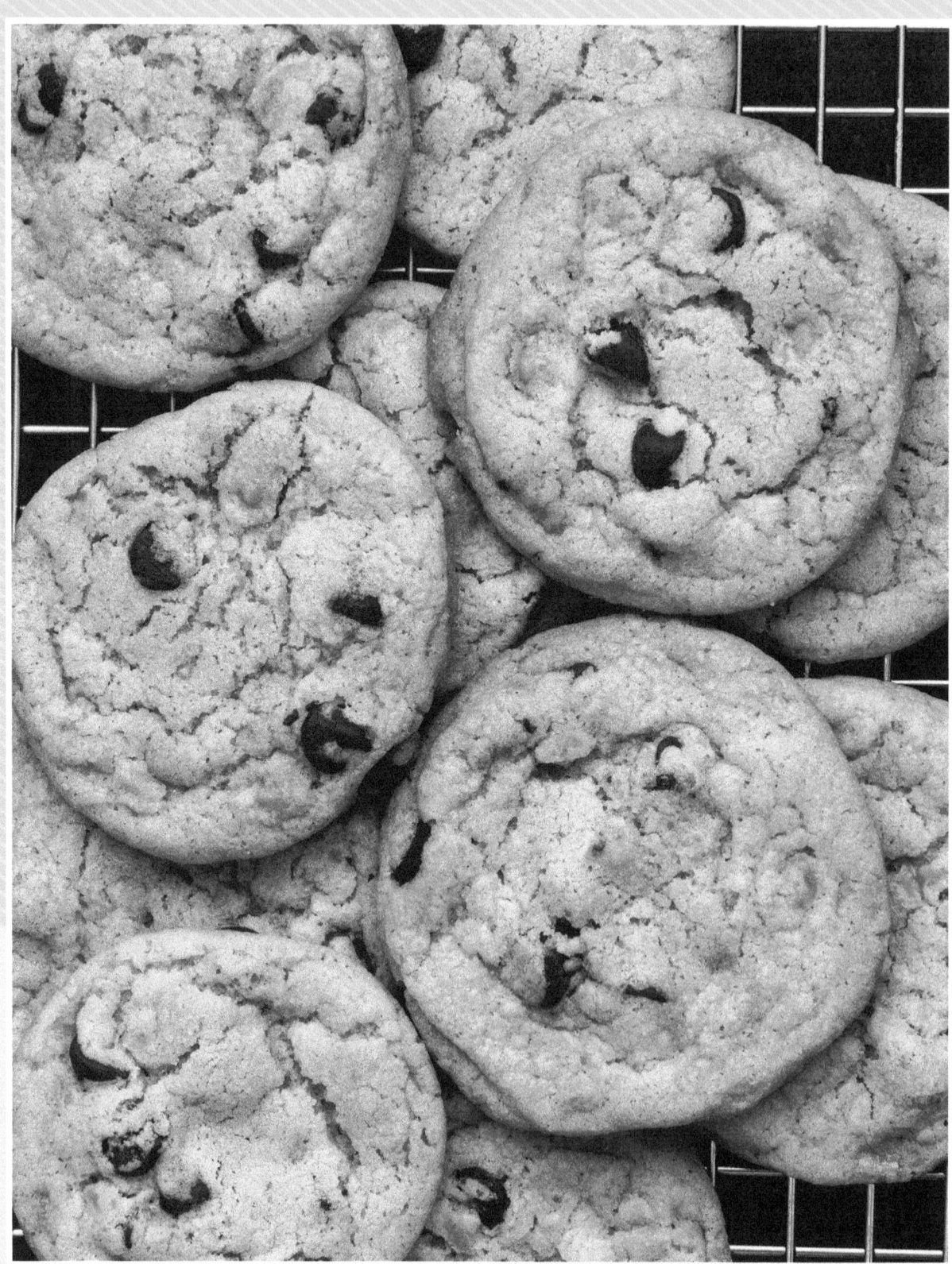

Chocolate Chunk Cookies, page 116.

CHAPTER 8

Sweet and Savory Baking

There are many types of baked goods, from cakes, muffins, and cookies to breads, pastries, and pies. In this chapter, you'll learn about sweet and savory baking. You'll also learn some essential techniques, such as how to make a piecrust, so that you, too, can offer to bring dessert next time you're invited somewhere.

Chocolate Chunk Cookies 116

Decadent Double Chocolate Brownies à la Mode 118

Cherry Lattice Pie 120

No-Brainer Banana Bread 123

Parmesan Herb Quick Bread 125

Tender Corn Bread 126

Rise Up

There is a lot of science that goes on during the baking process, which is why the process is much more precise than cooking. It's crucial to follow the ingredients, measurements, techniques, and temperatures so the recipe will turn out correctly. Recipes rely on ratios of ingredients. These ratios ensure that the recipe reacts appropriately with the heat.

Oven baking is the most common type of baking and is great for beginners. Oven baking uses dry heat in an enclosed space. The heat contacts the dough or batter and causes a reaction that results in color and texture changes.

SWEET AND SAVORY DOUGHS

Generally, there are two types of baked goods—sweet and savory. Sweet doughs include some sort of sweetener, such as sugar, honey, or maple syrup. Savory doughs get their flavor from other ingredients, such as herbs, spices, cheeses, or salt.

Typically, cakes and cookies come from sweet batters. Scones, pies, breads, and muffins can be either sweet or savory. For example, a blueberry pie is a sweet pie, whereas a ham-and-cheese quiche is a savory pie.

Most baked recipes use the same base ingredients—flour, a leavening agent, fat, salt, and dairy. Additional flavorings are added to the base to make the recipe unique. The techniques used to prepare the dough or batter also contribute to the finished baked good.

Prepping Baked Goods

When it comes to baking, success often lies in the preparation. Reading the recipe through before starting is especially important when baking. Before you start, you need to ensure you have the exact ingredients, at the proper temperature, if required.

I recommend measuring out all the ingredients before you start making the recipe. This technique is called "mise en place." It's a French term that means "everything in its place." This will ensure that you have the exact ingredients you need for the recipe and is a good overall practice for baking and cooking alike.

Baking is not the time to eyeball measurements. You need to measure all the ingredients provided in the recipe precisely. One tablespoon of baking powder does not mean 1 heaping tablespoon of baking powder. Dry ingredients should be scooped and then leveled off using a straight edge. See Measure it Out (page 9).

Using the proper ingredients—and not swapping them—is important in both savory and sweet baking. When a recipe calls for flour, it usually means all-purpose flour unless otherwise stated. Swapping whole wheat flour for all-purpose flour, for example, will not yield the same results because the structure of whole wheat flour is different. Similarly, baking powder and baking soda are two different leavening ingredients and cannot be used interchangeably.

Make sure the ingredients are fresh. This is very important for leavening agents like baking powder and yeast (check the expiration date on the package). Old, out-of-date ingredients can cause baked goods to turn out flat.

The last thing you need to consider is the preparation of the baking vessel. The recipe should indicate if you need to grease the pan. You can use nonstick cooking spray, butter, or shortening to grease a pan. Keep in mind, though; not all pans need to be greased. Refer to the recipe.

NOTES ON TIME, TEMPERATURE, AND COLOR

Temperature is critical when baking. If a recipe calls for room-temperature butter, you need to ensure you're not using butter straight from the refrigerator. Or, if a pie recipe calls for ice water, you need to use very cold water chilled with ice, not just cold tap water. These little details matter when baking. Unless the recipe specifically states otherwise, you should use room-temperature ingredients. The warmer temperature will help the ingredients combine more evenly. Plus, colder ingredients take longer to bake.

The temperature of the oven is also critical. As ovens get older, their temperature sensors can fail. I strongly recommend investing in an oven thermometer. This inexpensive gadget will tell you the temperature of the oven, regardless of the set temperature. This will allow you to see if the oven is running too cool or too hot, and you can adjust it as needed. When baking, it's important to keep the baking temperature consistent. Try to refrain from opening the oven door too often. Every time the door opens, the oven temperature will drop, resulting in uneven baking.

Sweet and Savory Baking

I recommend following the recipe baking time but with a little help from your senses to tell when the dish is almost done. When you start to really smell the baked good's aroma, that's a good indicator it's almost done. To check if a baked good is done, you can stick a toothpick into the center of the item and see if it comes out clean. If there is batter on the toothpick, it will need a little more bake time.

Color is another indicator of doneness. When baked items are light golden brown, they are usually done. The golden color actually creates a lot of flavor. Cakes will also start to pull away from the edges of the pan when they are done. When baked goods are finished baking, they need to be cooled. It's best to leave the item(s) in the pan or on the baking sheet and place the vessel on a cooling rack. This will allow airflow around the entire pan so it cools evenly. Most recipes will tell you how long to let something cool before removing it from the pan.

How to Cream Butter and Sugar

A recipe will often instruct you to "cream the butter and sugar." This means to mix softened butter and sugar at a fairly high speed until the butter and sugar are completely blended, fluffy, and pale yellow. It allows the sugar to dissolve into the butter and incorporates air into the batter.

BEST PRACTICES

It's important to use softened butter for this process. The easiest way to soften butter is to leave it on the counter for 8 hours before you plan to use it. Cold butter will not incorporate properly with the sugar, and butter that is too warm and soft will leave you with a greasy batter.

Cut the butter into cubes and add it to the mixing bowl. Add the sugar to the bowl, and set the mixer to medium speed (you can use a fork and a mixing spoon, but it will require a lot more elbow grease). As the mixture combines, you can increase the speed. The process will take about 5 minutes to get the desired consistency. Be sure to periodically stop the mixer and scrape down the sides of the bowl so all the sugar and butter is evenly combined.

TROUBLESHOOTING MISTAKES

Don't worry if you forgot to bring the butter to room temperature. There is an easy fix. Simply fill a microwave-safe measuring cup or bowl with water and microwave it on high for two minutes. Meanwhile, slice the butter into tablespoon-size pieces, and place it in an even layer on a heat-safe plate.

When the water is done, quickly remove the container from the microwave. But place the plate with the butter on it *in* the microwave and quickly close the door. In about 10 minutes, the leftover heat from the water will soften the butter.

How to Make Piecrust

Making a gorgeous, homemade piecrust that is golden and flaky is a win for any beginner baker. Piecrust has many uses for delicious sweet and savory dishes, such as pies, quiches, and potpies. The process is easy, and the ingredients are simple. It all comes down to technique and understanding what makes piecrust flaky and light.

BEST PRACTICES

Traditional pie dough is made by cutting fat into the flour until it looks like fine crumbs and adding ice water. The dough needs to chill for a while to allow the flour to hydrate fully. When the dough is rolled out, the fat stretches throughout the dough to form the layers. When those strands of butter in the dough melt during baking, forming steam and leaving behind air pockets, it results in flaky pie dough. The key is to keep the fat as solid as possible until the dough is baked so the steam and air pockets can form. If the fat melts before baking, the result is a tough, leathery dough.

Any type of heat during preparation is the nemesis of flaky pie dough. The easiest way to keep the fat from melting is to use ice-cold ingredients (keep the butter in the refrigerator until the last second) and not touch the dough with your hands. The heat from your hands, even the temperature of the room, can melt the fat. I like to make pie dough in a food processor to speed up the preparation process and ensure that I'm not touching and overworking the dough. Overworking it will also make tough pie dough.

TROUBLESHOOTING MISTAKES

Pie dough can easily stick to the work surface, making it difficult to transfer it to the pie dish. To alleviate this issue, after each roll, lift the dough and give it a quarter turn. This ensures that the dough is not sticking to the surface. Add a little more flour to the work surface if the dough starts to stick.

Pie dough can become tough if it's not kept cold. This is why it's important to work with cold ingredients. If you find that the dough is getting warm, return it to the refrigerator and allow it to chill.

If the dough tears when you transfer it to the pie dish, there's an easy fix. Simply press the tear together with your fingers. If the tear is too large to fix with your fingers, press a scrap of dough over the tear and press it into place.

Overworking the dough is another mistake that novice bakers make. Unfortunately, there's not much you can do at this point. Just chalk it up to experience and learn from it for next time.

How to Make Whipped Cream

Making whipped cream is a simple process that can make a big difference to desserts. Use it on pies, cakes, and baked goods. It's also an excellent topping for fresh fruit and other healthy treats. All you need is heavy whipping cream, vanilla, cream of tartar, and sugar to create the perfect dessert topping.

BEST PRACTICES

The fastest and easiest way to make whipped cream is to use an electric mixer on medium-high speed (you can whisk by hand; just keep the bowl cold). As you whip the cream, air gets trapped between the fat molecules in the cream, and it becomes light and fluffy. Whip the ingredients until soft peaks form. If you turn the whisk or beater upside down and a slight peak forms, it is done. The peak may droop a bit but should still hold its form. It should take about 5 minutes. Be careful not to whip the cream beyond this point, or it will begin turning into butter.

Whipped cream is very delicate. Adding cream of tartar to the recipe helps stabilize the whipped cream so it holds its shape longer. Cream of tartar is not a liquid, as the name implies. It's a dry powder found in the spice section of the grocery store.

TROUBLESHOOTING MISTAKES

When purchasing the cream for whipped cream, it's important to get heavy cream or whipping cream and not light cream. Heavy cream and whipping cream have a higher fat content and hold the shape longer.

With whipped cream, temperature matters. Not only should the tools and ingredients be cold, but hot weather can also cause whipped cream to wilt or melt. This is why we add cream of tartar to the mixture.

Chocolate Chunk Cookies

Makes 24 Cookies	**Prep time:** 15 minutes, plus 1 hour to chill, and time to cool completely	**Cook time:** 10 minutes per batch

Skills used: Measuring, creaming

- 1 cup (2 sticks) unsalted butter, at room temperature
- 1 cup granulated sugar
- 1 cup packed light brown sugar
- 2 large eggs
- 2 teaspoons pure vanilla extract
- 1 teaspoon baking soda
- 2 teaspoons hot water
- ½ teaspoon table salt
- 3 cups all-purpose flour
- 2 cups semisweet chocolate chunks or chips

Per Serving: Calories: 281; Fat: 14g; Saturated fat: 8g; Cholesterol: 37mg; Carbohydrates: 37g; Fiber: 2g; Protein: 3g; Sodium: 172mg

Everyone needs a go-to chocolate chip cookie recipe, because there is nothing more comforting, or anticipation-inducing, than the smell of chocolate chip cookies baking. These cookies are actually made with chocolate chunks, which give more chocolate flavor per bite, but you can also use chocolate chips if you prefer. To ensure the cookies bake evenly, they need to be a consistent size. You can use a tablespoon to measure the dough or use a cookie scoop.

1. In a large bowl, using a mixer on medium speed, cream together the butter, granulated sugar, and brown sugar until fluffy.

2. Turn the mixer speed down to low, and add the eggs one at a time, incorporating each egg into the mixture before adding the next. Stir in the vanilla.

3. In a small bowl, dissolve the baking soda into the hot water. This ensures that the baking soda will be equally distributed throughout the batter. Add this mixture to the batter, along with the salt, and stir to combine. Stir in the flour and chocolate chunks until just combined. You don't want to overmix the batter. Cover the dough, and chill it in the refrigerator for at least 1 hour or up to 24 hours.

4. Preheat the oven to 350°F. Line a baking sheet with parchment paper.

5. Scoop out 2-tablespoon dough dollops, and roll them into balls. Arrange 12 cookie dough balls on the prepared baking sheet.

6. Bake for 10 minutes, or until edges are lightly browned. Cool the cookies on the baking sheet for 5 minutes before transferring them to a cooling rack to cool completely. Repeat for the second batch.

7. To store leftovers, allow them to cool completely, place them in a container with a tight-fitting lid, and store at room temperature for up to 7 days.

VARIATION TIP: Take these cookies to the next level by stirring in 1 cup of chopped nuts, such as walnuts or pecans, or replace half the chocolate chunks with peanut butter chips.

TROUBLESHOOTING TIP: To prevent the cookies from spreading out too much when baking, make sure the baking sheets have time to cool between batches. Placing cookie dough on a hot baking sheet will make the cookies spread out more as they bake.

Decadent Double Chocolate Brownies à la Mode

Makes 16 Brownies	**Prep time:** 10 minutes, plus time to cool completely	**Cook time:** 45 minutes

Skills used: Measuring, sifting, whisking

It's no trouble to make brownies from scratch, especially when you see how much better they taste than the boxed versions. These fudgy brownies are super moist and just bursting with chocolate flavor. When you take them out of the oven, the center may be extra gooey, but as the brownies cool, they will continue to firm up to the perfect consistency. Serve with delicious homemade whipped cream.

FOR THE BROWNIES
Nonstick cooking spray
1½ cups granulated sugar
¾ cup all-purpose flour
¾ teaspoons table salt
⅔ cup natural, unsweetened cocoa powder (see Ingredient Tip)
½ cup confectioners' sugar
½ cup semisweet chocolate chips
2 large eggs
½ cup canola oil
2 tablespoons water
½ teaspoon pure vanilla extract
½ gallon (16 scoops) vanilla ice cream

FOR THE WHIPPED CREAM
1 cup heavy (whipping) cream, cold
½ teaspoon pure vanilla extract
¼ teaspoon cream of tartar
2 tablespoons confectioners' sugar

Per Serving: Calories: 401; Fat: 22g; Saturated fat: 10g; Cholesterol: 73mg; Carbohydrates: 48g; Fiber: 2g; Protein: 5g; Sodium: 178mg

1. Preheat the oven to 325°F. Line an 8-inch square baking dish with parchment paper and spray the parchment paper with cooking spray.
2. **To make the brownies:** In a medium bowl, combine the granulated sugar, flour, and salt. Sift in the cocoa powder and confectioners' sugar. Whisk together the dry ingredients until combined, then stir in the chocolate chips.

3. In a large bowl, combine the eggs, oil, water, and vanilla. Whisk until completely combined. Pour the dry ingredients into the wet ingredients, and stir until just combined. Be careful not to overmix the batter. Pour the batter into the prepared baking dish, and smooth the top with a spatula.

4. Bake for 45 minutes, or until a toothpick inserted into the center comes out with only a few crumbs attached. Cool the brownies completely before slicing. The time it takes to cool will vary depending on kitchen conditions. While you wait for them to cool, you can make the whipped cream.

5. **To make the whipped cream:** In a chilled bowl, combine the heavy cream, vanilla, and cream of tartar. Using an electric mixer or whisk, whip the mixture until the cream starts to change consistency. Add the confectioners' sugar, and continue whipping until medium peaks form.

6. Serve the cooled brownies with a scoop of vanilla ice cream and a dollop of whipped cream.

7. To store leftovers, allow the brownies to cool completely, place them in a container with a tight-fitting lid, and store at room temperature for up to 4 days. Store leftover whipped cream in a separate covered bowl in the refrigerator for up to 2 days.

INGREDIENT TIP: There are several types of cocoa powder available, including natural, Dutch process, and black. This recipe uses natural, unsweetened cocoa powder, which is the most common type. Natural cocoa is the powder that comes from roasted cocoa beans. It's bitter and quite acidic. It also has a strong chocolate flavor. Dutch process uses an alkaline solution that neutralizes the natural acid in the cocoa. It gives it a darker color and more mellow flavor. It also makes it easier to dissolve into liquids. Black cocoa is powder that has been heavily alkalized. It has a very dark brown color, almost black, and a strong flavor. It's usually used for its color and in combination with another type of cocoa powder.

Cherry Lattice Pie

Serves 8	**Prep time:** 1 hour, plus 1 hour to chill and 4 hours to cool	**Cook time:** 1 hour

Skills used: Measuring, mixing, making piecrust

Homemade cherry pie is an American classic. This recipe has a flavorful homemade filling enveloped in flaky piecrust. The recipe techniques are straightforward, and you can just follow along step-by-step, but you will need to plan for enough time to make the recipe. You can also make the dough and filling ahead of time and assemble and bake the pie later. Don't forget a dollop of whipped cream on top (see Decadent Double Chocolate Brownies à la Mode, page 118).

FOR THE DOUGH
- 2½ cups all-purpose flour, divided, plus more for the work surface
- 1 teaspoon table salt
- 1 tablespoon granulated sugar
- 1 cup (2 sticks) unsalted butter, very cold and cut into ½-inch cubes
- 6 tablespoons ice water, divided

FOR THE FILLING
- 4 cups fresh or frozen tart cherries, pitted, and halved (see Ingredient Tip)
- 1 cup granulated sugar
- ¼ cup cornstarch
- 1 tablespoon freshly squeezed lemon juice
- 1 teaspoon pure vanilla extract
- 1 tablespoon unsalted butter, cut into 6 small pieces

FOR THE EGG WASH
- 1 large egg
- 1 tablespoon whole milk

FOR THE WHIPPED CREAM
- 1 cup heavy (whipping) cream, cold
- ½ teaspoon pure vanilla extract
- ¼ teaspoon cream of tartar
- 2 tablespoons confectioners' sugar

Per Serving: Calories: 536; Fat: 26g; Saturated fat: 16g; Cholesterol: 88mg; Carbohydrates: 73g; Fiber: 3g; Protein: 6g; Sodium: 304mg

1. **To make the dough:** In the bowl of a food processor, combine 1½ cups of flour, the salt, and the sugar. Pulse it a few times until everything is combined. Add the butter cubes to the food processor, and pulse for about 15 seconds until the butter and flour are combined and the mixture looks grainy.

2. Scrape down the sides of the bowl, and add the remaining 1 cup of flour. Pulse until crumbly. Drizzle 4 tablespoons of ice water into the food processor, and pulse until the mixture starts coming together. If it's not forming a ball, add 2 more tablespoons of water, and pulse until the mixture forms a ball. Remove the dough from the bowl, and divide it in half. Flatten each portion into a disc shape, and wrap each in plastic wrap. Refrigerate for at least 1 hour or for up to 2 days.

3. **To make the filling:** In a large bowl, combine the cherries, sugar, cornstarch, lemon juice, and vanilla. Stir until thoroughly combined. Cover the bowl with plastic wrap, and refrigerate for at least 30 minutes or up to 24 hours.

4. Remove one disc of chilled pie dough from the refrigerator, and allow it to come to room temperature for 5 minutes. Lightly flour the work surface, the rolling pin, and the top of the dough. Roll the dough into a 12-inch circle that is ⅛ inch thick. Transfer the dough to a 9-inch pie dish, and gently press it in.

5. Use a slotted spoon to transfer the chilled cherries from the bowl to the pie dish. Reserve the juice in the bowl. Refrigerate the pie as you work on the next step.

6. In a small saucepan, heat 3 tablespoons of the reserved cherry juice over medium-high heat until it reduces and is slightly thick. Allow the juice to cool for 5 minutes, and drizzle it over the cherries in the piecrust. Arrange the 6 small butter pieces on top of the cherries.

7. Preheat the oven to 400°F.

8. Remove the remaining disc of dough from the refrigerator, and lightly flour the work surface, the rolling pin, and the top of the dough. Roll the dough into a 12-inch circle that is ⅛ inch thick. Use a sharp knife to cut the dough into ½-inch-thick strips.

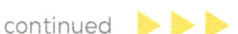

continued

Cherry Lattice Pie continued

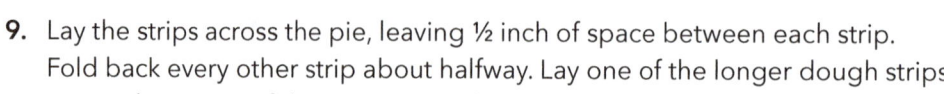

9. Lay the strips across the pie, leaving ½ inch of space between each strip. Fold back every other strip about halfway. Lay one of the longer dough strips across the center of the pie on top of the remaining strips.

10. Unfold the strips that were pulled back, and lay them across the long dough strip you just placed. Fold back the strips that were not pulled back previously. Lay another dough strip across the pie about ½ inch from the previous strip. Repeat this process until the pie is latticed.

11. Trim the edges of the lattice dough so that it's flush with the bottom layer of dough. Fold the bottom layer of pie dough over the lattice strips around the edges. Crimp the dough to secure it.

12. **To make the egg wash:** In a small bowl, whisk together the egg and milk until fully combined. Brush the egg wash over the top of the pie.

13. Place the pie on a rimmed baking sheet, and bake for 20 minutes. Reduce the oven heat to 375°F, and bake for an additional 35 minutes or until the crust is golden brown and the filling is bubbling. Remove the pie from the oven, and allow it to cool completely, about 4 hours.

14. When cooled, slice the pie, and serve it with dollops of whipped cream, if you'd like.

15. To store leftovers, cover the pie, and refrigerate it for up to 5 days.

INGREDIENT TIP: If using frozen cherries, be sure to thaw them completely before using. If using fresh cherries, you can easily remove the pits with a chopstick. Place the chopstick into the top, indented end of the cherry, and push it through, forcing the pit out of the opposite end.

No-Brainer Banana Bread

Makes 2 loaves	Prep time: 15 minutes, plus 40 minutes to cool	Cook time: 1 hour

Skills used: Measuring, beating

Nonstick cooking spray
3 cups all-purpose flour, plus more for dusting pan
12 tablespoons (1½ sticks) unsalted butter, at room temperature
1 (8-ounce) package cream cheese, at room temperature
2 cups granulated sugar
½ teaspoon pure vanilla extract
2 large eggs
½ teaspoon baking powder
½ teaspoon baking soda
½ teaspoon table salt
1½ cups mashed bananas (from 4 medium bananas)

Per Serving (⅛ loaf): Calories: 335; Fat: 14g; Saturated fat: 8g; Cholesterol: 62mg; Carbohydrates: 48g; Fiber: 1g; Protein: 4g; Sodium: 186mg

This banana bread recipe is the perfect way to use up overripe bananas that are about to go bad. In fact, this recipe works best with bananas that are past their prime, because the bananas are sweeter and have a stronger banana flavor. This easy-breezy recipe works well for dessert or for a grab-and-go breakfast.

1. Preheat the oven to 350°F. Spray 2 (8-by-4-inch) loaf pans with cooking spray, and lightly dust them with flour.

2. In a large bowl, beat the butter and cream cheese with an electric (or stand) mixer until creamy. Slowly add the sugar and vanilla, beating until light and fluffy. Add the eggs one at a time, beating between each addition until fully incorporated. In a medium bowl, stir together 3 cups of flour, the baking powder, the baking soda, and the salt.

3. While the mixer is on low, slowly add the flour mixture to the cream cheese mixture until just combined. Stir in the mashed bananas with a rubber spatula.

4. Divide the batter evenly between the two prepared loaf pans. Bake them for 1 hour or until a toothpick inserted into the center of each loaf comes out clean. To prevent over-browning, you may need to cover the loaves with aluminum foil for the last 15 minutes of baking.

continued ▶▶▶

No-Brainer Banana Bread continued

5. Cool the loaves in the pan for 10 minutes. Remove them from the pans, and then cool them on a wire rack for an additional 30 minutes before slicing.

6. To store leftovers, allow the bread to cool completely, wrap it tightly with plastic wrap, and store at room temperature for up to 3 days.

VARIATION TIP: For a delicious twist, add chocolate chips to this recipe. In a small bowl, stir together 1 cup of semisweet chocolate chops with ¼ cup of additional all-purpose flour. Pour the coated chocolate chips into the batter in step 4, and fold in. Continue with the recipe as directed.

Parmesan Herb Quick Bread

Makes 10 to 12 slices	Prep time: 15 minutes, plus time to cool completely	Cook time: 50 minutes

Skills used: Measuring, whisking

Nonstick cooking spray
3 cups all-purpose flour
½ cup grated Parmesan cheese
3 tablespoons granulated sugar
1 tablespoon baking powder
½ teaspoon dried rosemary
½ teaspoon dried thyme
½ teaspoon table salt
1 large egg
1 cup whole milk
5⅓ tablespoons (½ stick plus 1⅓ tablespoons) unsalted butter, melted and slightly cooled

Per Serving: Calories: 249; Fat: 9g; Saturated fat: 5g; Cholesterol: 42mg; Carbohydrates: 35g; Fiber: 1g; Protein: 7g; Sodium: 382mg

This flavorful bread isn't made with yeast. Instead, the bread gets its rise from the baking powder, so there's no need to knead. The texture of quick breads is more like a muffin than a bread. Enjoy it for breakfast with a little touch of butter, or use it to sop up the juices of a delicious dinner, such as Simple Scrumptious Shrimp Scampi (page 64).

1. Preheat the oven to 350°F. Spray an 8-by-4-inch loaf pan with cooking spray.

2. In a large bowl, combine the flour, Parmesan cheese, sugar, baking powder, rosemary, thyme, and salt. Whisk together, and make a well, or an indent, in the center of the mixture.

3. In a medium bowl, whisk together the egg, milk, and butter. Pour the wet ingredients into the well in the dry ingredients. Stir together until just combined.

4. Pour the batter into the prepared loaf pan, and bake for 40 to 50 minutes, or until a toothpick inserted into the center comes out clean. Cool the bread in the pan for 10 minutes. Remove the bread from the pan and continue to cool on a wire rack.

5. To store leftovers, allow it to cool completely, wrap it tightly with plastic wrap, and store at room temperature for up to 2 days. You can also freeze it for up to 3 months. To freeze, slice the bread first.

Tender Corn Bread

Serves 9	**Prep time:** 10 minutes	**Cook time:** 18 minutes

Skills used: Whisking, measuring

Nonstick cooking spray
1 cup yellow cornmeal
½ cup all-purpose flour
1 tablespoon baking powder
1 teaspoon table salt
½ teaspoon baking soda
1 large egg
1 cup buttermilk
½ cup milk
¼ cup canola oil

Per Serving: Calories: 177; Fat: 8g; Saturated fat: 1g; Cholesterol: 25mg; Carbohydrates: 21g: Fiber: 1g; Protein: 4g; Sodium: 493mg

Corn bread is a cake-like quick bread made from cornmeal instead of entirely from flour. This is a great beginner recipe, because corn bread doesn't get its life from yeast. The baking powder reacts with the acidic buttermilk to make it fluffy and tender. Buttermilk tends to separate as it sits, though, so shake it well before measuring it. Serve this corn bread warm with a bit of butter or drizzled with honey for a bit of sweetness. It pairs perfectly with the No-Sweat Three-Bean Chili (page 34).

1. Preheat the oven to 450°F. Spray an 8-inch square baking dish with cooking spray and set aside.

2. In a small bowl, whisk the cornmeal, flour, baking powder, salt, and baking soda until combined.

3. In a medium bowl, whisk the egg, buttermilk, milk, and oil until fully combined. Add the dry ingredients to the wet ingredients, and stir until just combined. Be careful not to overmix the batter.

4. Transfer it to the prepared baking dish, and bake for 15 to 18 minutes, or until a toothpick inserted in the center comes out clean.

5. To store leftovers, allow the corn bread to cool completely, tightly wrap it with plastic wrap, and store it at room temperature for up to 2 days.

FLAVOR BOOST: Like it spicy? Kick up the heat by adding a jalapeño pepper. Remove the stem, seeds, and rib from the jalapeño, and finely mince it. Stir it into the batter in step 3.

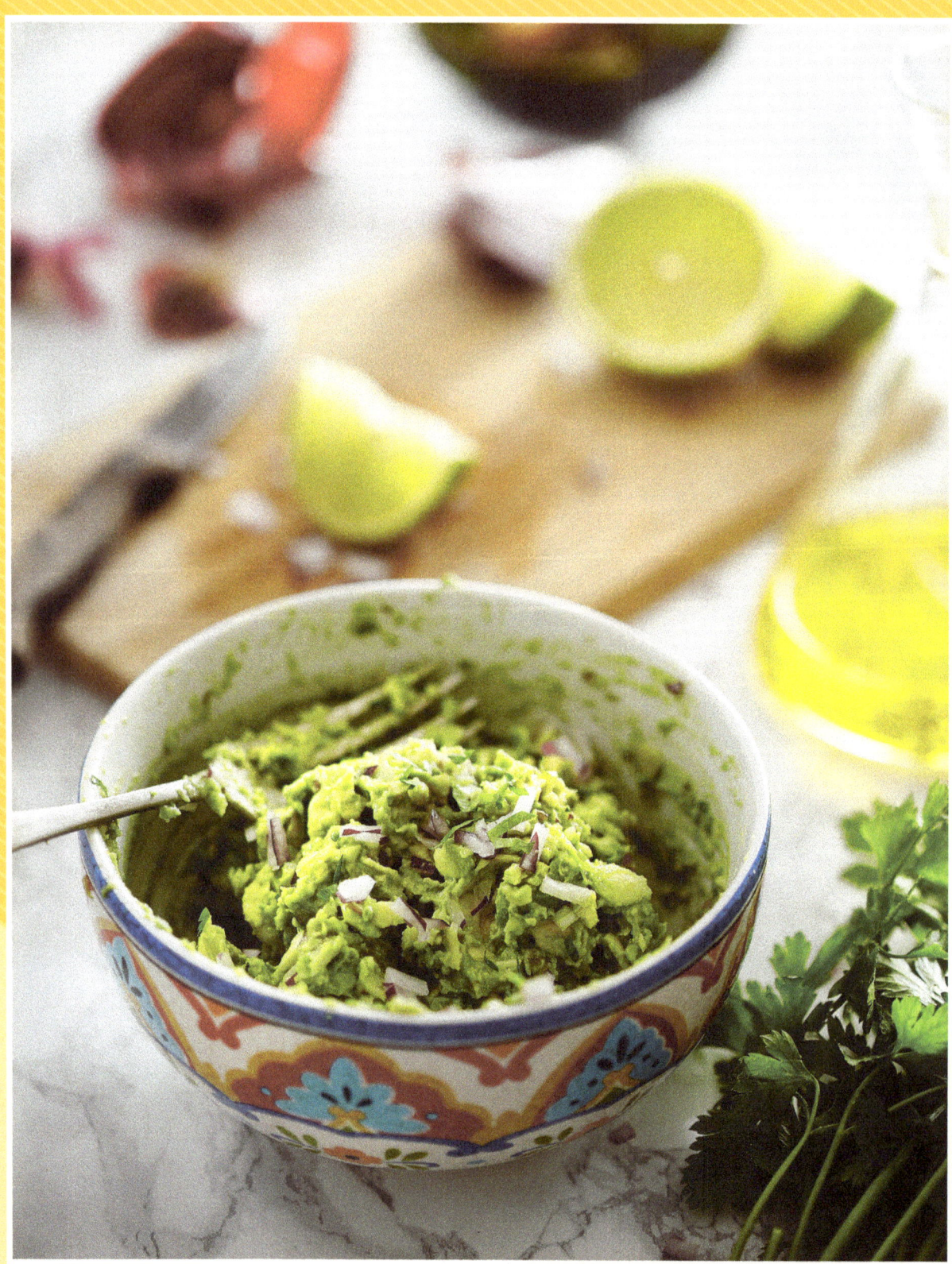

Classic Guacamole, page 130.

CHAPTER 9

Recipes That Bring It All Together

This chapter has a selection of recipes that allow you to practice the various skills you've learned to this point. It's an opportunity to put your newfound knowledge to the test and further develop your skills. I've included classic recipes that, as you get more confident, you can adapt to suit your tastes.

Classic Guacamole 130

Easy-Peasy Pasta Salad 131

Citrus-Glazed Fruit Salad 132

Pancakes with Blueberry Compote
and Lemon Whipped Cream 134

Mini Veggie Frittatas 136

Balsamic Roasted Brussels Sprouts 137

Baked Macaroni and Cheese 138

Spicy Roasted Chicken Legs 140

Sunday Pot Roast 142

Classic Guacamole

Serves 4	Prep time: 10 minutes

Skills used: Knife skills, measuring, pitting avocado

- 3 ripe avocados
- 2 Roma tomatoes, chopped
- ½ cup red onion, finely diced
- 1 garlic clove, minced
- 1 jalapeño pepper, seeded and finely diced
- 3 tablespoons chopped fresh cilantro
- Juice from 1 lime
- 1 teaspoon table salt
- ¼ teaspoon cayenne pepper

Per Serving: Calories: 266; Fat: 22g; Saturated fat: 3g; Cholesterol: 0mg; Carbohydrates: 19g; Fiber: 11g; Protein: 4g; Sodium: 597mg

Avocados can be intimidating if you've never worked with them. But with these tips, it's actually quite easy and kind of fun to pit and peel. To remove the flesh from an avocado, use a chef's knife to cut into the avocado until you hit the pit. Run a knife lengthwise around the entire avocado, cutting down to the pit. Once you've cut all the way around, gently twist both halves of the avocado in opposite directions to release one half from the pit. Use a spoon to carefully remove the pit, then scrape the flesh of the avocado into the bowl.

1. Remove the flesh and pit the avocados. In a medium bowl, mash the avocado flesh with a fork. If you like your guacamole chunky, stop mashing while there are still some larger chunks of avocado left. If you prefer a smoother texture, keep mashing until you reach the desired consistency.

2. Stir in the tomatoes, onion, garlic, jalapeño, cilantro, lime juice, salt, and cayenne. Serve immediately.

3. To store leftovers, place a layer of plastic wrap directly onto the guacamole, and gently press it down. Refrigerate for 1 day.

SUBSTITUTION TIP: This guac is easy to make, but if you want to take a shortcut, replace the chopped tomatoes, diced onion, and minced garlic with 1½ cups of prepared pico de gallo.

Easy-Peasy Pasta Salad

| Serves 6 | **Prep time:** 20 minutes | **Cook time:** 10 minutes |

Skills used: Knife skills, measuring, cooking pasta

3 cups dry rotini pasta

¼ cup plus 1 tablespoon extra-virgin olive oil, divided

3 tablespoons freshly squeezed lemon juice (from 1 lemon)

3 garlic cloves, minced

1 teaspoon Dijon mustard

1 teaspoon Italian seasoning

¾ teaspoon table salt

¼ teaspoon red pepper flakes

2 cups halved cherry tomatoes

1 (15-ounce) can chickpeas, drained and rinsed

1 cup quartered cucumber slices

1 cup sliced black olives

½ cup minced fresh parsley

1 cup crumbled feta cheese

Per Serving: Calories: 471; Fat: 21g; Saturated fat: 6g; Cholesterol: 22mg; Carbohydrates: 57g; Fiber: 7g; Protein: 15g; Sodium: 706mg

This pasta salad has a bright, lemony dressing. Adding the dressing to the warm noodles allows the pasta to absorb the flavors of the dressing, making for a more flavorful salad. This dish can be enjoyed as a main with a side such as Balsamic Roasted Brussels Sprouts (page 137) or can be a side to a wonderful main dish such as Perfect Roast Chicken (page 86).

1. Bring a large pot of salted water to a boil. Add the pasta, and cook according to the package directions. Drain the pasta, and place it in a large bowl. Add 1 tablespoon olive oil, and toss until the pasta is coated.

2. While the pasta cooks, in a small container with a tight-fitting lid, combine ¼ cup of olive oil with the juice, garlic, mustard, Italian seasoning, salt, and red pepper flakes. Affix the lid, and shake until fully combined.

3. To the large bowl with the pasta, add the cherry tomatoes, chickpeas, cucumbers, black olives, and parsley. Stir until all the ingredients are thoroughly combined. Pour the dressing over the pasta, and toss until everything is evenly coated. The warm pasta absorbs the dressing more easily, creating a more flavorful pasta salad. Stir in the feta cheese just before serving.

4. To store leftovers, place them in a container with a tight-fitting lid, and refrigerate for up to 3 days.

Citrus-Glazed Fruit Salad

Serves 6	**Prep time:** 25 minutes, plus 3 hours to chill and time to cool	**Cook time:** 10 minutes

Skills used: Knife skills, measuring, zesting

2 navel oranges
1 lime
⅔ cup orange juice
⅓ cup pineapple juice
⅓ cup honey
1 teaspoon pure vanilla extract
3 bananas, sliced
2 cups chopped fresh pineapple
2 cups strawberries, hulled and sliced
2 cups blueberries
1 cup seedless grapes, halved

Per Serving: Calories: 248; Fat: 1g; Saturated fat: 0g; Cholesterol: 0mg; Carbohydrates: 64g; Fiber: 6g; Protein: 3g; Sodium: 5mg

Fruit salad is a beautiful and easy way to eat healthy, and is a nice dish to bring for a party or potluck. There are so many delicious fruits available year-round allowing you to customize the flavors of this recipe to suit your tastes. You can even prepare them to a theme: tropical, or citrus-centered, or berry blast. The bright citrus glaze here gives the salad a sweet tang.

1. Zest the oranges to yield ½ teaspoon orange zest. Put the orange zest in a medium saucepan. Reserve the oranges.

2. Zest the lime to yield ½ teaspoon lime zest and add the zest to the saucepan. Slice the zested lime in half, and squeeze the juice into a sieve placed over the saucepan.

3. Add the orange juice, pineapple juice, and honey to the saucepan, and turn the heat to medium-high. Bring to a boil, then reduce the heat to medium-low and simmer for 5 minutes.

4. Remove the sauce from the heat and stir in the vanilla. Allow it to cool completely.

5. Peel the reserved oranges and chop them into ½-inch pieces. Put them in a large bowl. To the same bowl, add the bananas, pineapple, strawberries, blueberries, and grapes.

6. Pour the cooled sauce over the fruit, and toss until all of the fruit is coated in the sauce.

7. Cover and refrigerate the fruit salad for 3 hours before serving.

8. To store leftovers, place the fruit salad in a container with a tight-fitting lid, and refrigerate for up to 2 days.

FLAVOR BOOST TIP: Give this fruit salad a minty flavor by adding 2 to 3 tablespoons of chopped fresh mint leaves to the sauce in step 1.

Pancakes with Blueberry Compote and Lemon Whipped Cream

Serves 4	**Prep time:** 15 minutes	**Cook time:** 15 minutes

Skills used: Measuring, whisking

Who can resist pancakes? Everyone should have their own homemade recipe. So, here is yours, and it's a good one. These pancakes are bright and decadent; I mean, they do have lemon whipped cream, after all. You can get a head start on this recipe by making the blueberry compote 1 day ahead of time. When you're ready to serve it, bring it to a simmer in a saucepan over medium heat to reheat it.

FOR THE BLUEBERRY COMPOTE

1 pint fresh blueberries
¼ cup water
2 tablespoons honey
1 teaspoon freshly squeezed lemon juice

FOR THE PANCAKES

1 cup all-purpose flour
2 tablespoons granulated sugar
2 tablespoons baking powder
½ teaspoon table salt
1 cup half-and-half
1 large egg
2 tablespoons canola oil
1 teaspoon pure vanilla extract
Nonstick cooking spray

FOR THE WHIPPED CREAM

1 cup cold heavy (whipping) cream
½ teaspoon pure vanilla extract
¼ teaspoon cream of tartar
2 tablespoons confectioners' sugar
1 tablespoon lemon zest
1 teaspoon freshly squeezed lemon juice

Per Serving: Calories: 579; Fat: 38g; Saturated fat: 19g; Cholesterol: 150mg; Carbohydrates: 55g; Fiber: 2g; Protein: 8g; Sodium: 902mg

1. **To make the blueberry compote:** In a small saucepan, heat the blueberries, water, and honey over medium heat, and bring to a simmer. Simmer for 7 minutes or until the sauce thickens, stirring occasionally. Transfer the sauce to a large bowl, and stir in the lemon juice. Set aside.

2. **To make the pancakes:** In a large bowl, combine the flour, granulated sugar, baking powder, and salt; stir to combine. In a small bowl, combine the half-and-half, egg, oil, and vanilla. Whisk together until the egg is fully combined. Whisk the wet ingredients into the dry ingredients until just combined. The batter may be lumpy.

3. Preheat a griddle or large nonstick skillet over medium-high heat, and spray with cooking spray. Use a ¼-cup scoop to pour batter onto the hot griddle (you may have to work in batches). Cook for 2 to 3 minutes or until bubbles rise to the top of the pancakes. Flip the pancakes, and cook for another 2 to 3 minutes, or until bottoms are lightly browned. Remove them to a plate and cover with aluminum foil. Continue with the remaining batter, spraying the pan with additional cooking spray as necessary.

4. **To make the whipped cream:** In a chilled bowl, combine the heavy cream, vanilla, and cream of tartar. Using an electric mixer or whisk, whip the mixture until the cream starts to change consistency. Add confectioners' sugar, and continue whipping until medium peaks form. Fold the lemon zest and juice into the prepared whipped cream.

5. To serve, top the pancakes with warmed-up blueberry compote and lemon whipped cream.

6. To store leftovers, allow everything to cool completely, place pancakes in a zip-top bag, and store them the refrigerator for up to 3 days. Store the blueberry compote in a container with a tight-fitting lid and refrigerate for up to 3 days. Store the whipped cream in a container with a tight-fitting lid and refrigerate for up to 2 days.

GENERAL TIP: Make a double batch of the pancakes and freeze half of them for another time. Place cooled pancakes in a zip-top freezer bag and freeze for up to one month. To reheat, place frozen pancakes in a single layer on a rimmed baking sheet and bake in a 350°F preheated oven for 10 minutes.

Mini Veggie Frittatas

| Serves 6 | **Prep time:** 15 minutes | **Cook time:** 30 minutes |

Skills used: Knife skills, measuring, sautéing

Nonstick cooking spray
1 tablespoon extra-virgin olive oil
1 cup chopped white button mushrooms
¼ cup chopped green bell pepper
2 tablespoons chopped red onion
6 large eggs
½ cup whole milk
¼ teaspoon table salt
⅛ teaspoon freshly ground black pepper
1 cup shredded cheddar cheese

Per Serving: Calories: 185; Fat: 14g; Saturated fat: 6g; Cholesterol: 207mg; Carbohydrates: 3g; Fiber: 0g; Protein: 12g; Sodium: 299mg

These frittatas make an excellent, healthy grab-and-go breakfast for busy mornings. Or make them as a fun brunch treat to serve friends along with Pancakes with Blueberry Compote and Lemon Whipped Cream (page 134) or Citrus-Glazed Fruit Salad (page 132). To reheat cold frittatas, loosely wrap a frittata in a damp paper towel and microwave on high for 20-second intervals until heated through.

1. Preheat the oven to 350°F. Spray a 12-cup muffin pan with cooking spray.

2. In a 10- to 12-inch skillet, heat the oil over medium heat until shimmering. Add the mushrooms, bell pepper, and onion to the skillet; sauté for 5 to 10 minutes. The mushrooms and peppers should be fork-tender.

3. In a medium bowl, whisk the eggs, milk, salt, and pepper until they are fully combined and no streaks of egg are visible. Stir the cooked vegetables and cheddar cheese into the egg mixture.

4. Using a ¼-cup scoop, fill each muffin cup. Bake for 20 minutes or until the eggs are set, and the edges are lightly browned.

5. To store leftovers, allow them to cool completely, place them in a container with a tight-fitting lid, and refrigerate for up to 3 days.

SUBSTITUTION TIP: Lighten up this recipe by swapping the whole eggs for 12 egg whites or 1½ cups of egg substitute. Replace the whole milk with skim milk or your favorite nondairy substitute.

Balsamic Roasted Brussels Sprouts

| Serves 4 | **Prep time:** 10 minutes | **Cook time:** 25 minutes |

Skills used: Knife skills, measuring, sautéing, roasting

- 1 tablespoon extra-virgin olive oil
- 2 tablespoons unsalted butter
- 1½ pounds Brussels sprouts, trimmed, halved, stem end and loose outer leaves removed
- ¾ teaspoon table salt
- ½ teaspoon freshly ground black pepper
- 1 garlic clove, minced
- 1 tablespoon balsamic vinegar

Per Serving: Calories: 159; Fat: 10g; Saturated fat: 4g; Cholesterol: 15mg; Carbohydrates: 16g; Fiber: 7g; Protein: 6g; Sodium: 480mg

Brussels sprouts look like tiny cabbages because they are members of the cabbage family. Not only are they good for you—they are an excellent source of vitamins C and K, fiber, and iron among many other nutrients—but when roasted, the natural sweetness and crisp texture may steal the show. These sprouts are a great side dish to serve with Perfect Roast Chicken (page 86) or Sunday Pot Roast (page 142).

1. Preheat the oven to 425°F.
2. Heat a 10- or 12-inch oven-safe skillet over medium-high heat. Combine the olive oil and butter in the skillet. When the butter has melted, add the Brussels sprouts. Season with the salt and pepper.
3. Allow the sprouts to brown on one side, 2 to 3 minutes. Turn them over, stir in the minced garlic, brown for 1 to 2 minutes, and transfer the skillet to the oven.
4. Roast for 10 to 15 minutes, or until the sprouts are tender and golden brown.
5. Carefully remove the skillet from the oven, and toss the sprouts with the balsamic vinegar.
6. To store leftovers, allow the sprouts to cool completely, place them in a container with a tight-fitting lid, and refrigerate for up to 3 days.

INGREDIENT TIP: Whenever you are cooking or roasting vegetables, they should all be cut to a similar size so they cook evenly.

Baked Macaroni and Cheese

| Serves 4 | **Prep time:** 15 minutes | **Cook time:** 25 minutes |

Skills used: Knife skills, measuring, cooking pasta

¼ cup unsalted butter, plus more for greasing
2 cups dried elbow pasta
¼ cup all-purpose flour
¾ cup whole milk
1¼ cups half-and-half
2 cups grated medium sharp cheddar cheese, divided
1 cup grated Gruyère cheese, divided
1 teaspoon table salt
½ teaspoon freshly ground black pepper

Per Serving: Calories: 792; Fat: 50g; Saturated fat: 30g; Cholesterol: 150mg; Carbohydrates: 51g; Fiber: 2g; Protein: 33g; Sodium: 1,083mg

Macaroni and cheese is pure comfort food and a true crowd pleaser. I like using Gruyère cheese, because it melts perfectly and has a slightly salty flavor that cuts through some of the richness. For a creamier cheese sauce, swap 1 cup of cheddar cheese for 1 cup of processed American cheese cut into ½ inch cubes.

1. Preheat the oven to 325°F. Grease an 8-inch square baking dish with butter.

2. Bring a large pot of salted water to a boil over medium-high heat. When the water is boiling, add the pasta, and cook for 1 minute less than the package directions, about 8 to 11 minutes. Drain the pasta, and set aside.

3. While the pasta water is boiling, in a large saucepan, melt the butter over medium heat. When the butter has melted, whisk in the flour for 1 minute. Slowly pour in the milk while whisking constantly until smooth. Pour in the half-and-half, and whisk until it's combined and smooth. Continue whisking for 1 to 2 minutes, until the mixture thickens. You can tell when it's thick enough by placing a spoon into the mixture, lifting it out, and running your finger down the back of the spoon. If it leaves a line on the spoon, it's the perfect consistency.

4. Turn off the heat, and add 1½ cups of cheddar cheese, ¾ cups of Gruyère cheese, the salt, and the pepper. Stir until they are melted and completely combined. Now stir in the cooked pasta.

5. Transfer it to the prepared baking dish, and top with the remaining ½ cup of cheddar cheese and ¼ cup of Gruyère cheese. Bake for 15 minutes, until the cheese bubbles and becomes a light, golden brown.

6. To store leftovers, allow the casserole to cool completely, cover it with a tight-fitting lid, and refrigerate for up to 4 days.

VARIATION TIP: You can turn this side dish into a complete meal by adding 2 cups of cooked shredded or chopped chicken and 1 cup of steamed broccoli florets during step 5.

Spicy Roasted Chicken Legs

| Serves 4 | **Prep time:** 10 minutes | **Cook time:** 35 minutes |

Skills used: Knife skills, measuring, roasting

Nonstick cooking spray
1 teaspoon table salt
½ teaspoon garlic powder
½ teaspoon onion powder
¼ teaspoon freshly ground black pepper
8 chicken legs, patted dry
¼ cup unsalted butter
Juice from 1 lemon
2 garlic cloves, minced
½ teaspoon sriracha
¼ teaspoon cayenne pepper

Per Serving: Calories: 595; Fat: 47g; Saturated fat: 17g; Cholesterol: 241mg; Carbohydrates: 2g; Fiber: 0g; Protein: 38g; Sodium: 774mg

Now this is an easy dinner that you won't want to miss. Don't skimp on the butter, because it helps the chicken legs stay moist and juicy. If you prefer a crisper skin, when the chicken is done cooking, move the baking sheet to the top oven rack, and turn on the broiler. Broil the chicken until the skin reaches the desired crispness. Don't walk away from the broiler; the chicken can burn quickly.

1. Preheat the oven to 450°F. Line a rimmed baking sheet with aluminum foil and spray it with cooking spray.

2. In a small bowl, combine the salt, garlic powder, onion powder, and pepper. Season both sides of the chicken legs with the salt mixture.

3. In a small saucepan, melt the butter over medium-high heat. When the butter has melted, add the lemon juice, garlic, sriracha, and cayenne, and stir to combine. Reserve 3 tablespoons of the butter mixture, and set it aside.

4. Using tongs, dip the chicken legs into the butter mixture, ensuring that each piece is completely coated. Place the coated chicken on the prepared baking sheet.

5. Bake for 30 to 35 minutes. During the last 5 minutes of baking, brush the chicken with the reserved butter mixture. The chicken is done when it's golden brown and has reached an internal temperature of 165° F.

6. To store leftovers, allow the legs to cool completely, place them in a container with a tight-fitting lid, and refrigerate for up to 3 days.

VARIATION TIP: If you prefer your chicken less spicy, swap the cayenne for chili powder, which is milder. You can also replace the sriracha with sweet chili sauce, which has a sweet, garlicky flavor.

Sunday Pot Roast

Serves 4	**Prep time:** 10 minutes	**Cook time:** 3 hours 10 minutes

Skills used: Knife skills, measuring

1 (3- to 5-pound) beef chuck roast

2 teaspoons table salt, divided

1 teaspoon freshly ground black pepper, divided

2 tablespoons canola oil

3 garlic cloves, sliced

1 cup red wine (see Ingredient Tip)

2 cups low-sodium beef broth

2 tablespoons Worcestershire sauce

2 yellow onions, cut into 1-inch pieces

1 pound baby carrots

1 pound baby red potatoes, halved

3 sprigs fresh thyme

2 sprigs fresh rosemary

Per Serving: Calories: 865; Fat: 49g; Saturated fat: 19g; Cholesterol: 225mg; Carbohydrates: 36g; Fiber: 6g; Protein: 69g; Sodium: 871mg

This Sunday pot roast is not just reserved for 1950s sitcoms. This beef is fall-apart tender, and the sauce is rich and flavorful. I grew up just loving this recipe. It is straightforward to make, but it does require several hours of hands-off cooking time. Serve this roast with Mashed Potatoes in a Snap (page 52) and Balsamic Roasted Brussels Sprouts (page 137) or Robust Roasted Root Vegetables (page 53).

1. Preheat the oven to 325° F.

2. Season all sides of the chuck roast with 1 teaspoon salt and ½ teaspoon pepper. In an oven-safe Dutch oven, heat the canola oil over medium-high heat. When the oil is shimmering, add the chuck roast and sear until the bottom is golden brown, 1 to 2 minutes per side. Repeat until all sides are seared to a golden brown. Transfer the chuck roast to a plate.

3. Now add the garlic to the Dutch oven, and cook for 30 seconds. Pour in the red wine, and scrape up any bits on the bottom of the pan. After 3 to 5 minutes, when the wine has reduced by about half, add the roast back to the Dutch oven.

4. Add the beef broth, Worcestershire sauce, onions, carrots, potatoes, thyme, and rosemary. Season with the remaining 1 teaspoon salt and ½ teaspoon pepper, put the lid on the Dutch oven, and immediately transfer it to the preheated oven.

5. Cook for 3 hours or until the roast reaches an internal temperature of 200°F and pulls apart easily with a fork. Remove it from the oven, and slice it with the grain. It may be so tender that it falls apart.

6. To store leftovers, allow the roast to cool completely, place it in a container with a tight-fitting lid, and refrigerate for up to three days.

INGREDIENT TIP: Use a full-bodied red wine, such as a merlot or cabernet sauvignon, in this recipe. Or, if you prefer to not use wine at all, substitute an extra cup of low-sodium beef broth in place of the wine.

GENERAL TIP: Use the leftovers to make an open-faced roast beef sandwich. Reheat 1½ cups of shredded beef with ½ cup of sauce in a saucepan. Place 2 slices of hearty sandwich bread on a plate and top the bread with the warmed beef and sauce.

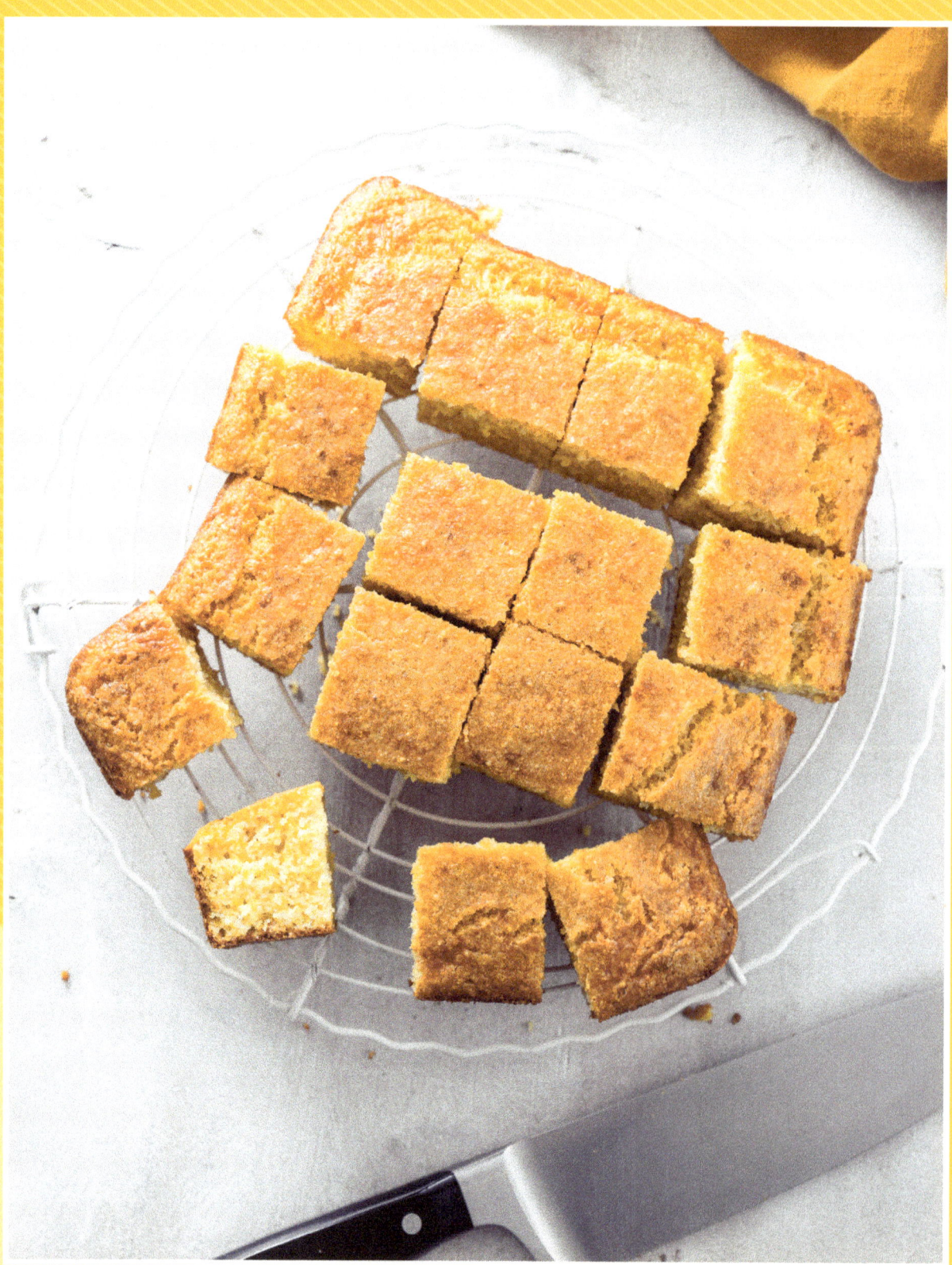

Tender Corn Bread, page 126.

Measurements and Conversions

—

VOLUME EQUIVALENTS	U.S. STANDARD	U.S. STANDARD (OUNCES)	METRIC (APPROXIMATE)
LIQUID	2 tablespoons	1 fl. oz.	30 mL
	¼ cup	2 fl. oz.	60 mL
	½ cup	4 fl. oz.	120 mL
	1 cup	8 fl. oz.	240 mL
	1½ cups	12 fl. oz.	355 mL
	2 cups or 1 pint	16 fl. oz.	475 mL
	4 cups or 1 quart	32 fl. oz.	1 L
	1 gallon	128 fl. oz.	4 L
DRY	⅛ teaspoon	–	0.5 mL
	¼ teaspoon	–	1 mL
	½ teaspoon	–	2 mL
	¾ teaspoon	–	4 mL
	1 teaspoon	–	5 mL
	1 tablespoon	–	15 mL
	¼ cup	–	59 mL
	⅓ cup	–	79 mL
	½ cup	–	118 mL
	⅔ cup	–	156 mL
	¾ cup	–	177 mL
	1 cup	–	235 mL
	2 cups or 1 pint	–	475 mL
	3 cups	–	700 mL
	4 cups or 1 quart	–	1 L
	½ gallon	–	2 L
	1 gallon	–	4 L

OVEN TEMPERATURES

FAHRENHEIT	CELSIUS (APPROXIMATE)
250°F	120°C
300°F	150°C
325°F	165°C
350°F	180°C
375°F	190°C
400°F	200°C
425°F	220°C
450°F	230°C

WEIGHT EQUIVALENTS

U.S. STANDARD	METRIC (APPROXIMATE)
½ ounce	15 g
1 ounce	30 g
2 ounces	60 g
4 ounces	115 g
8 ounces	225 g
12 ounces	340 g
16 ounces or 1 pound	455 g

Resources

AmericanLamb.com: For information regarding lamb, including quality, preparation, and recipes.

Beef.org: For information regarding beef, including quality, preparation, and recipes.

CDC.gov/healthyweight/healthy_eating/portion_size.html: For information on appropriate portion sizes.

ItIsaKeeper.com: This is my site! Here, you'll find easy recipes using easy-to-find-ingredients.

MyPlate.gov: For information on a nutritious and balanced diet.

Nutrition.gov: To learn about making healthy eating choices.

Pork.org: For information regarding pork, including quality, preparation and recipes.

USDA.gov: For comprehensive nutrition and food safety resources.

Index

A
Apples
  coring, 48
  Easy as Apple Crisp, 55
Apricot Miso Pork Tenderloin, 102-103

B
Bacon
  cooking, 96
  Grilled Bacon Cheeseburger, 98-99
  Velvety Pasta Carbonara, 40-41
Baked goods, 110-112. *See also* Desserts
Baking, 11
Baking dishes, 4
Baking sheets, rimmed, 4
Balanced meals, 19-20
Balsamic Roasted Brussels Sprouts, 137
Banana Bread, No-Brainer, 123-124
Beans
  about, 29
  No-Sweat Three-Bean Chili, 34-35
  prepping, 30
  soaking and cooking, 32-33
  troubleshooting, 33
Beef
  about, 92-93
  cooking ground, 97
  Easy-Breezy Beef Tacos, 100-101
  Grilled Bacon Cheeseburger, 98-99
  prepping, 94
  slicing against the grain, 95
  Sunday Pot Roast, 142-143
Bitter flavors, 17, 18
Blueberry Compote and Lemon Whipped Cream, Pancakes with, 134-135
Boiling, 10
Braising, 11
Breads
  No-Brainer Banana Bread, 123-124
  Parmesan Herb Quick Bread, 125
  Tender Corn Bread, 126
Broiling, 11
Brownies à la Mode, Decadent Double Chocolate, 118-119
Brussels Sprouts, Balsamic Roasted, 137
Burn prevention, 8

C
Can openers, 2
Carbohydrates, 19
Cheese
  Baked Macaroni and Cheese, 138-139
  Grilled Bacon Cheeseburger, 98-99
  Parmesan Herb Quick Bread, 125
  Velvety Pasta Carbonara, 40-41
Cherry Lattice Pie, 120-122
Chicken
  about, 74
  carving, 78-79
  Chicken Cutlets with Lemony Pan Sauce, 80-81
  cutlets, pounding, 77-78
  Perfect Roast Chicken, 86-87
  prepping, 76
  Sheet-Pan Chicken Shawarma, 84-85
  Soothing Chicken Noodle Soup, 82-83
  Spicy Roasted Chicken Legs, 140-141
Chili, No-Sweat Three-Bean, 34-35
Chocolate
  Chocolate Chunk Cookies, 116-117
  Decadent Double Chocolate Brownies à la Mode, 118-119

Chopping, 6
Citrus-Glazed Fruit Salad, 132-133
Coconut Curry Salmon, 70-71
Colanders, 2
Convection ovens, 12
Cookies, Chocolate Chunk, 116-117
Cooktops, 13
Corn Bread, Tender, 126
Creaming butter and sugar, 112-113
Cross contamination, 8
Curry Salmon, Coconut, 70-71
Cutting boards, 2

D

Denver Omelet, 88-89
Desserts
   Cherry Lattice Pie, 120-122
   Chocolate Chunk Cookies, 116-117
   Decadent Double Chocolate
      Brownies à la Mode, 118-119
   Easy as Apple Crisp, 55
Dicing, 6
Doughs, 110
Dutch ovens, 4

E

Eggs
   about, 75
   Denver Omelet, 88-89
   Mini Veggie Frittatas, 136
   omelets, 76-77

F

Fats, 19-20
Fire extinguishers, 8
Fish and seafood
   about, 58-60
   Coconut Curry Salmon, 70-71
   cooking in foil packets, 62-63
   Lemon Butter Fish Packets, 68-69
   prepping, 60-61
   Simple Scrumptious Shrimp Scampi, 64-65
   Soy-Ginger Scallops, 67
   Sticky Honey Garlic Shrimp, 66
   thawing frozen, 61
Flavor
   balancing with texture, 17-19
   basic tastes, 16-17
   developing, 16
Food processors, 5
Fresh staples, 21-22
Frittatas, Mini Veggie, 136
Frozen staples, 22
Fruits. *See also specific*
   about, 46
   Citrus-Glazed Fruit Salad, 132-133
   prepping, 47-48
Frying pans, 5

G

Garlic
   Garlic and Herb Lamb
      Chops, 106-107
   mincing, 49-50
   Sticky Honey Garlic Shrimp, 66
Ginger Scallops, Soy-, 67
Grains, 28
Grilling, 10
Grocery shopping tips, 24
Guacamole, Classic, 130

H

Hand mixers, electric, 5
Hand washing, 8
Herbs, 22-23
   Garlic and Herb Lamb
      Chops, 106-107
   Parmesan Herb Quick Bread, 125
Honey Garlic Shrimp, Sticky, 66

I

Immersion blenders, 5
Ingredient staples
   fresh, 21-22
   frozen, 22
   pantry, 20-21

K

Kettles, electric, 5
Kitchen shears, 2
Knife sharpener, 5
Knife skills, 6-7
Knives, 3

L

Lamb
  about, 93-94
  Garlic and Herb Lamb Chops, 106-107
  prepping, 94
  slicing against the grain, 95
Legumes, 29, 30
Lemons
  Chicken Cutlets with Lemony Pan Sauce, 80-81
  Lemon Butter Fish Packets, 68-69
  Pancakes with Blueberry Compote and Lemon Whipped Cream, 134-135

M

Macaroni and Cheese, Baked, 138-139
Macronutrients, 19
Measuring cups and spoons, 3
Measuring ingredients, 9
Meats, 92. *See also* Beef; Lamb; Pork
Meat tenderizers, 3
Meat thermometers, 3
Micronutrients, 19
Microwaves, 5
Mincing, 7
Miso Pork Tenderloin, Apricot, 102-103
Mixing bowls, 4
Multi-cookers, 5
Mustard Pan Sauce, Skillet Pork Chops with, 104-105

N

Noodles. *See* Pasta and noodles
Nutrition, 19-20

O

Onions, cutting, 48-49
Ovens, 12

P

Pancakes with Blueberry Compote and Lemon Whipped Cream, 134-135
Panfrying, 11
Pantry staples, 20-21
Parmesan Herb Quick Bread, 125
Pasta and noodles
  about, 28-29
  Baked Macaroni and Cheese, 138-139
  cooking, 30
  Easy-Peasy Pasta Salad, 131
  prepping, 30
  Simple Scrumptious Shrimp Scampi, 64-65
  Soothing Chicken Noodle Soup, 82-83
  troubleshooting, 31
  Veggie Ramen Bowl, 42
  Velvety Pasta Carbonara, 40-41
Peeling, 7
Pie, Cherry Lattice, 120-122
Piecrusts, 113-114
Pie dishes, 4
Pork. *See also* Bacon
  about, 94
  Apricot Miso Pork Tenderloin, 102-103
  prepping, 94
  Skillet Pork Chops with Mustard Pan Sauce, 104-105
  slicing against the grain, 95
Portion control, 20
Potatoes
  Mashed Potatoes in a Snap, 52
  Robust Roasted Root Vegetables, 53
Pot Roast, Sunday, 142-143
Poultry. *See* Chicken; Turkey
Preparing to cook, 13
Proteins, 19

R

Ramen Bowl, Veggie, 42
Recipes
  about, 25
  reading, 9

Rice
  about, 28
  cooking, 31–32
  Creamy Risotto, 36–37
  prepping, 30
  Simple Rice Pilaf, 38–39
  troubleshooting, 32
Rice cookers, 5
Roasting, 10

S

Safety tips, 8
Salads
  Citrus-Glazed Fruit Salad, 132–133
  Classic Tossed Salad with Homemade Vinaigrette, 51
  Easy-Peasy Pasta Salad, 131
Salmon, Coconut Curry, 70–71
Salty flavors, 16, 18
Saucepans, 5
Sautéing, 11
Scallops, Soy-Ginger, 67
Seafood. *See* Fish and seafood
Searing, 11
Seasoning, 17
Shawarma, Sheet-Pan Chicken, 84–85
Shellfish, 59. *See also* Fish and seafood
Shrimp
  peeling and deveining, 62
  Simple Scrumptious Shrimp Scampi, 64–65
  Sticky Honey Garlic Shrimp, 66
Simmering, 10
Skillets, 5
Slicing, 7
Soups
  Soothing Chicken Noodle Soup, 82–83
  Veggie Ramen Bowl, 42
Sour flavors, 17, 18
Soy-Ginger Scallops, 67
Spatulas, 3
Spices, 22–23
Spoons, 3
Steaming, 10
Stir-Fry, Rainbow, 54
Stir-frying, 11
Stoves, 13
Sunday Pot Roast, 142–143
Sweet flavors, 16, 18

T

Tacos, Easy-Breezy Beef, 100–101
Taste profiles, 16–17, 18
Textures, 17–19
Tongs, 4
Turkey
  about, 75
  carving, 78–79
  prepping, 76

U

Umami flavors, 17, 18

V

Vegetable peelers, 4
Vegetables. *See also specific*
  about, 46–47
  Classic Tossed Salad with Homemade Vinaigrette, 51
  Mini Veggie Frittatas, 136
  prepping, 47–48
  Rainbow Stir-Fry, 54
  Robust Roasted Root Vegetables, 53
  Veggie Ramen Bowl, 42
Vinaigrette, Classic Tossed Salad with Homemade, 51

W

Whipped cream, 114–115
  Decadent Double Chocolate Brownies à la Mode, 118–119
  Pancakes with Blueberry Compote and Lemon Whipped Cream, 134–135
Whisks, 4

Acknowledgments

To Mom and Dad for always encouraging us to follow our dreams. I wouldn't be who I am today without your support.

To my grandmothers, my mother-in-law, and Aunt Tina, who always had time to take me under their wings in the kitchen. I'll always remember the lessons you taught me and cherish every recipe and memory.

To the Callisto team, thank you for your guidance in bringing this book to life.

And, as always, to Jim and Joe. My faithful taste testers and daily support system. I love you!

About the Author

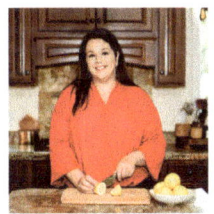

Christina Hitchcock is the creator and owner of the popular food blog *It Is a Keeper* (ItIsAKeeper.com). Her passion is sharing quick and easy recipes for busy families using easy-to-find, everyday ingredients. Christina discovered her love for cooking by spending time with her grandmothers in the kitchen. Her award-winning recipes have been featured on television, in national magazines, and on numerous online sites. Christina lives in Northeast Pennsylvania with her husband and son. Follow her on Facebook (@itsakeeper), Instagram, YouTube, Twitter, and Pinterest (@itsakeeperblog).

www.ingramcontent.com/pod-product-compliance
Lightning Source LLC
LaVergne TN
LVHW070948070426
835507LV00029B/3456